YOUNG
VOICES

YOUNG VOICES

Life with Diabetes

Author: Hala Khalaf

Editor: Markela Dedopoulos

Photographer: Jesper Westley

Art Director & Graphic Designer: Morten Agergaard

Special thanks to Karina Porcelli and Charlotte Ersbøll.

Published by Novo Nordisk A/S

in association with John Wiley & Sons Ltd.

January 2005

Novo Nordisk A/S

Novo Allé

2880 Bagsværd

DENMARK

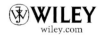

Distributed by Wiley

John Wiley & Sons Ltd.

The Atrium

Southern Gate, Chichester

West Sussex PO 19 8SQ, England

Printed and bound by Narayana Press, Denmark

ISBN 0 470 01584 5

YOUNG VOICES

Author
Hala Khalaf

Photographer
Jesper Westley

novo nordisk®

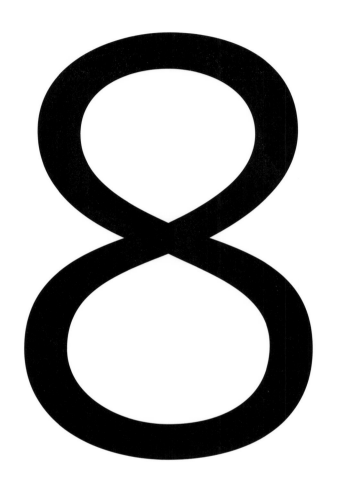

Stories

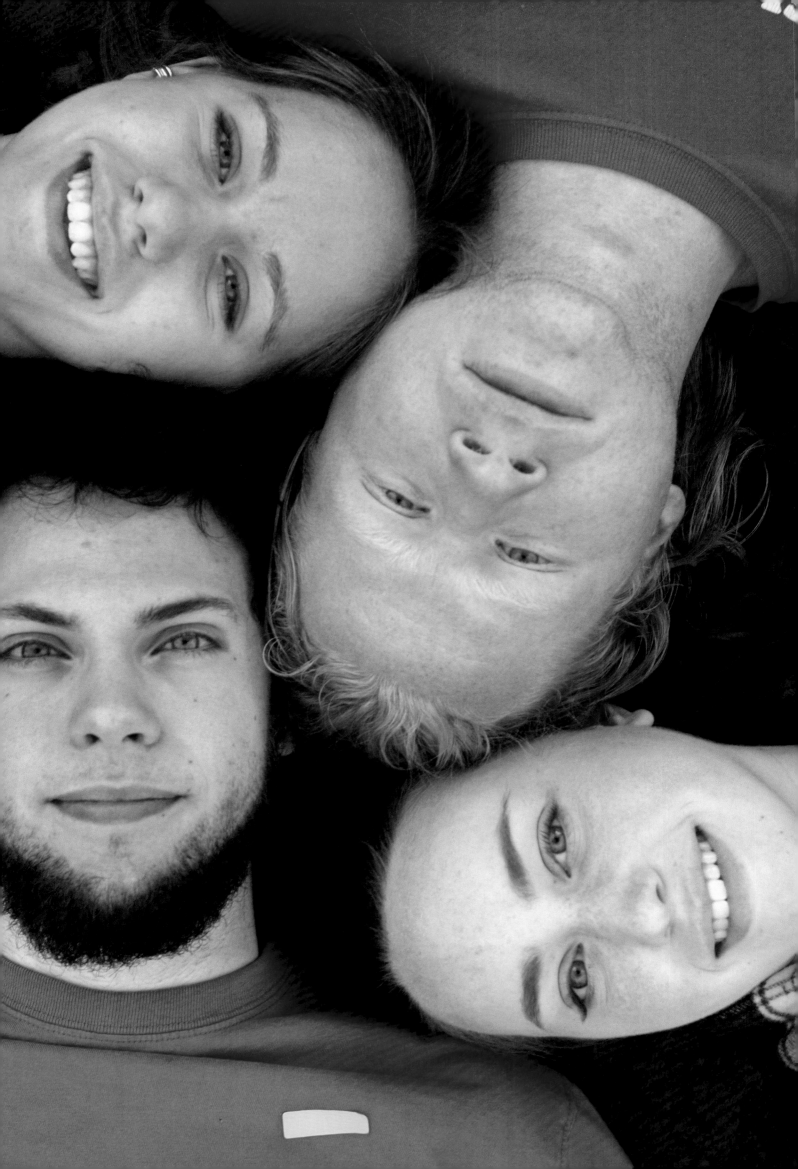

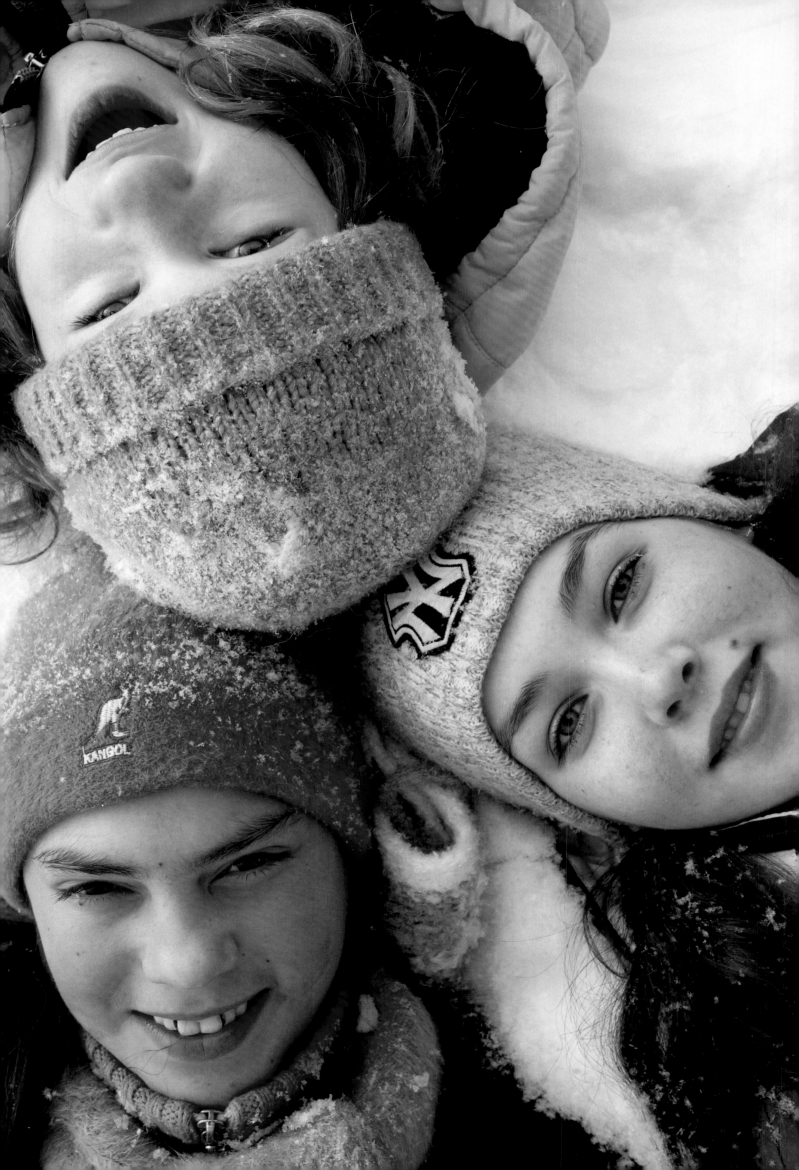

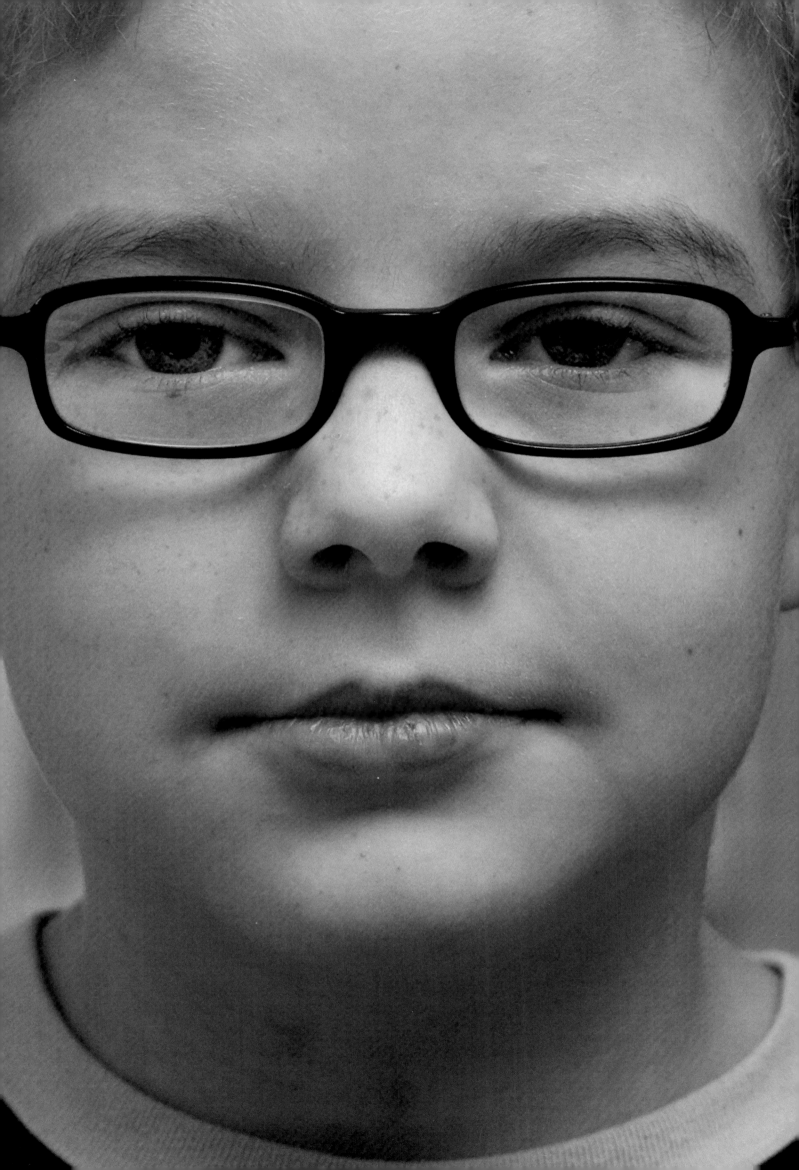

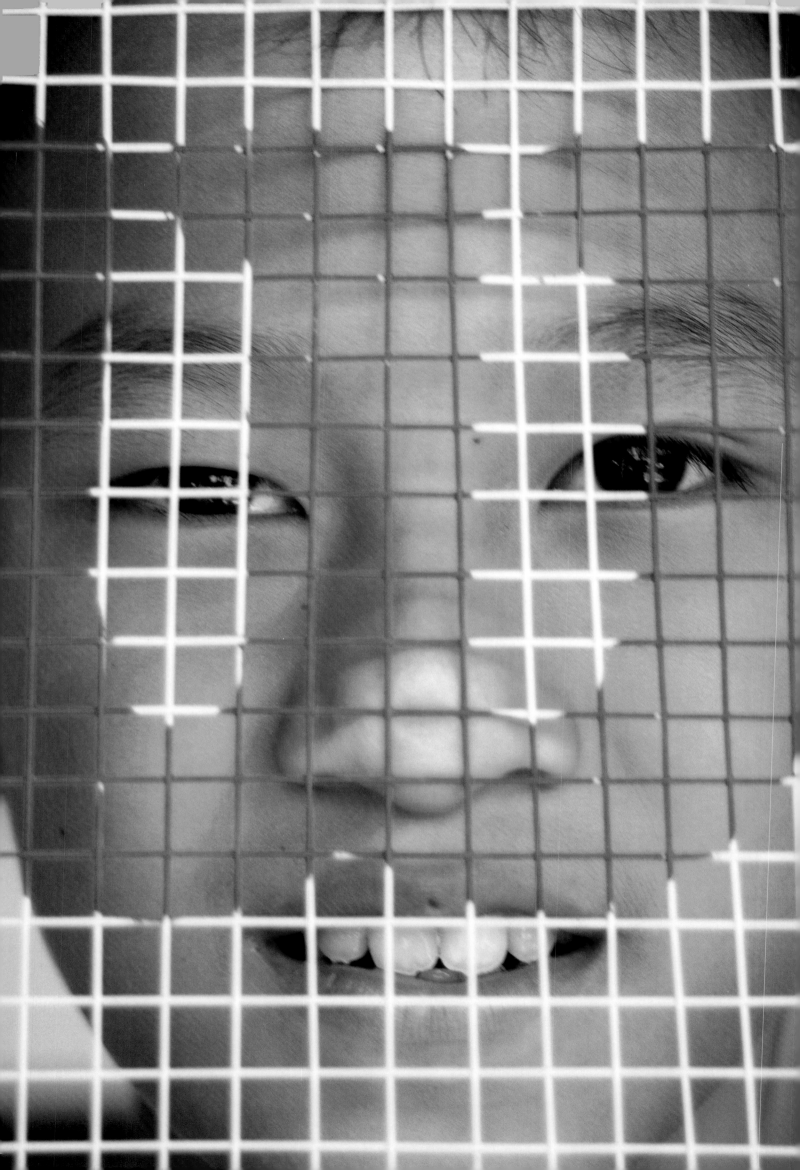

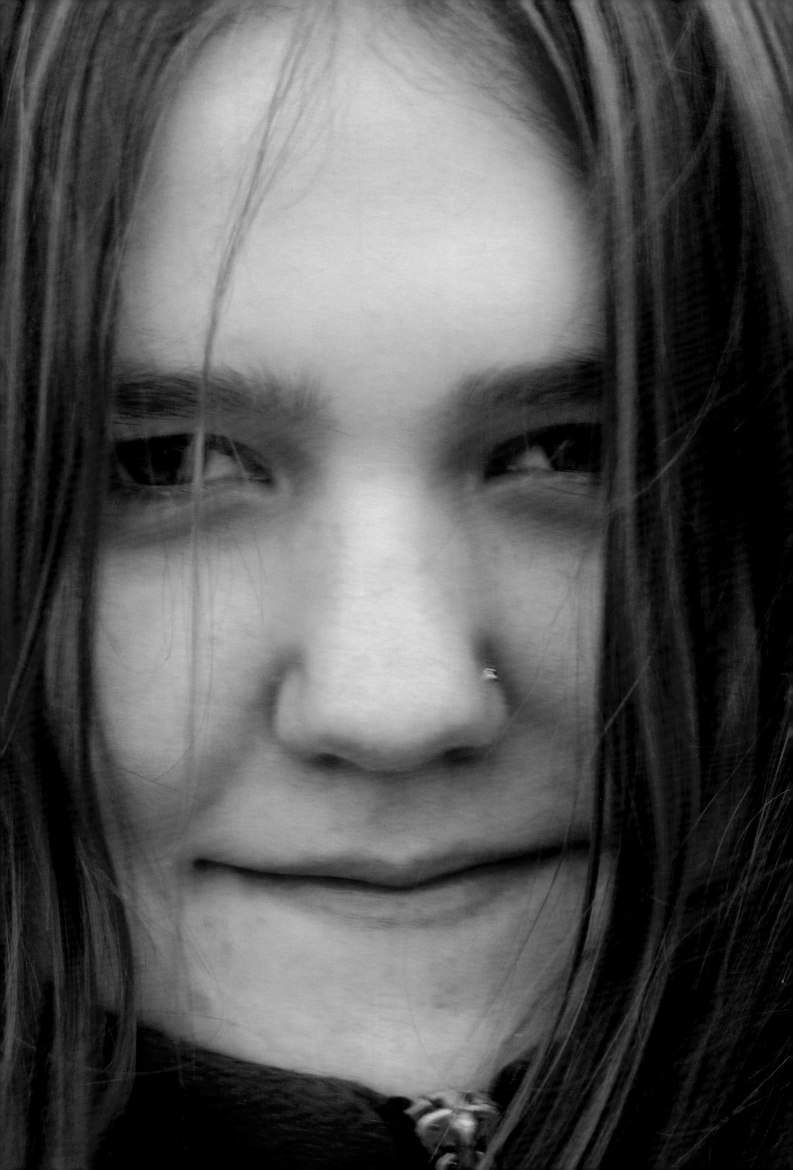

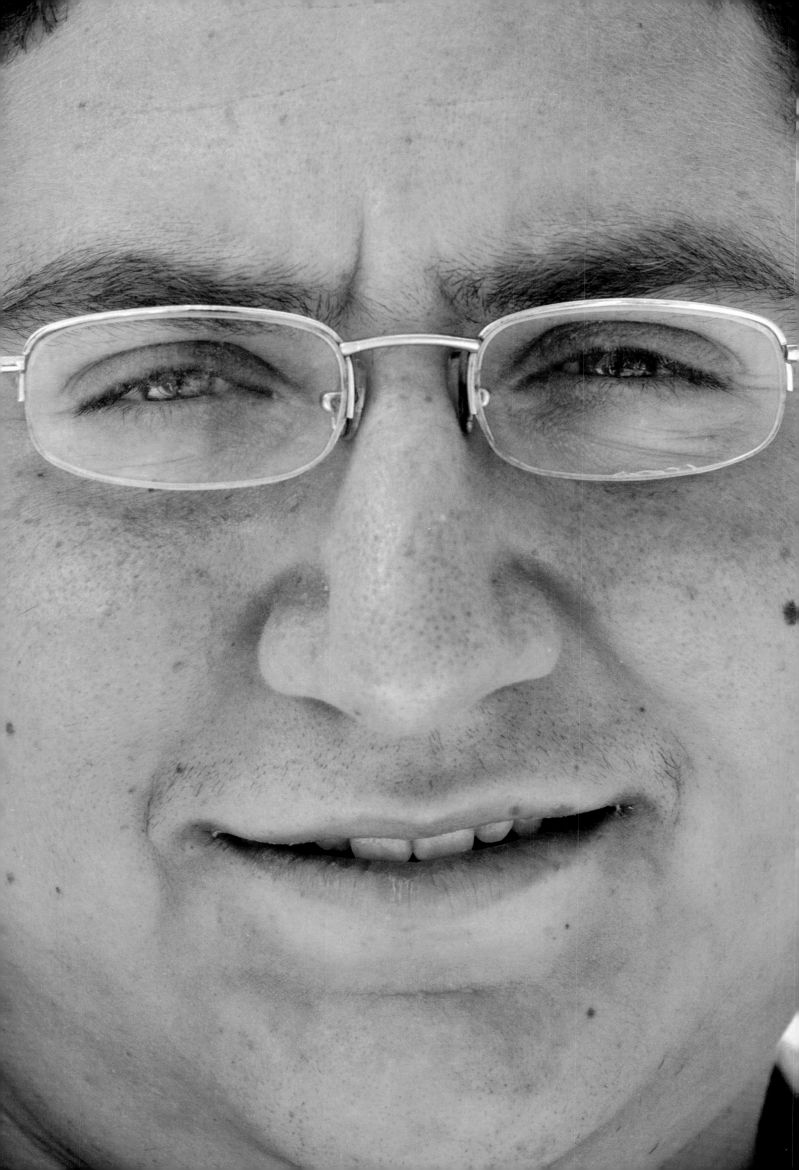

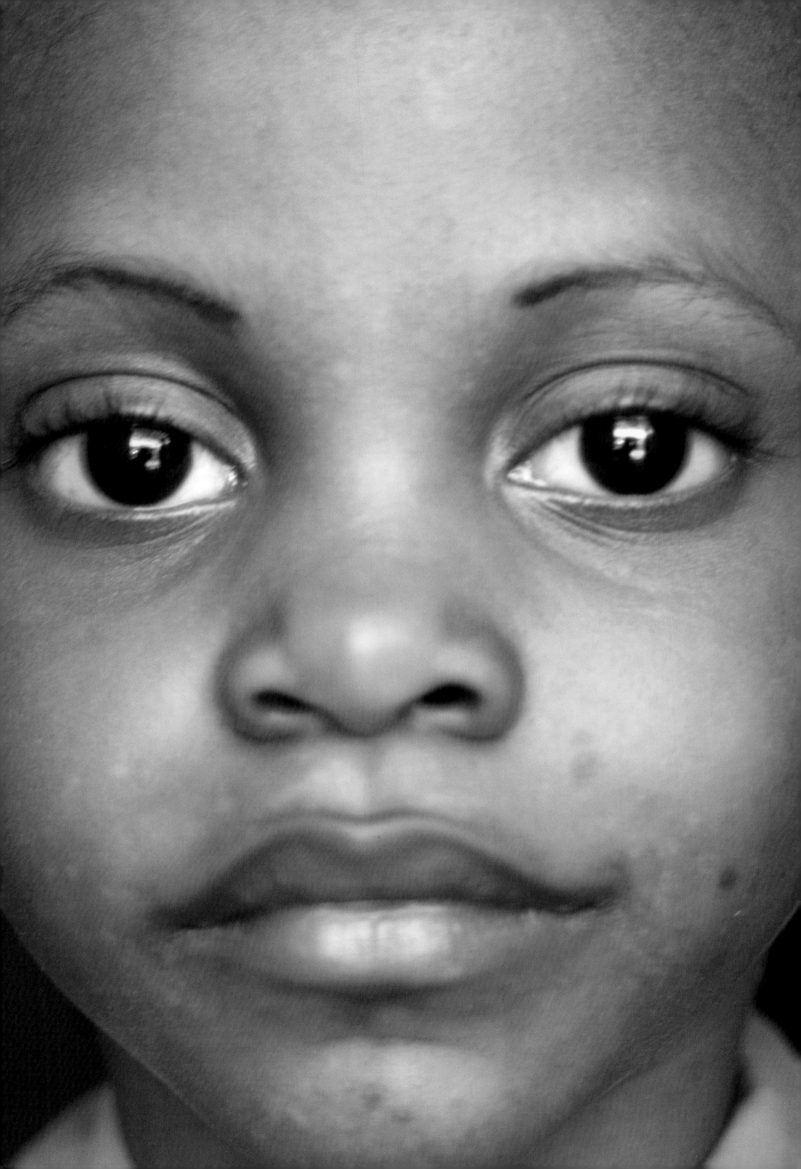

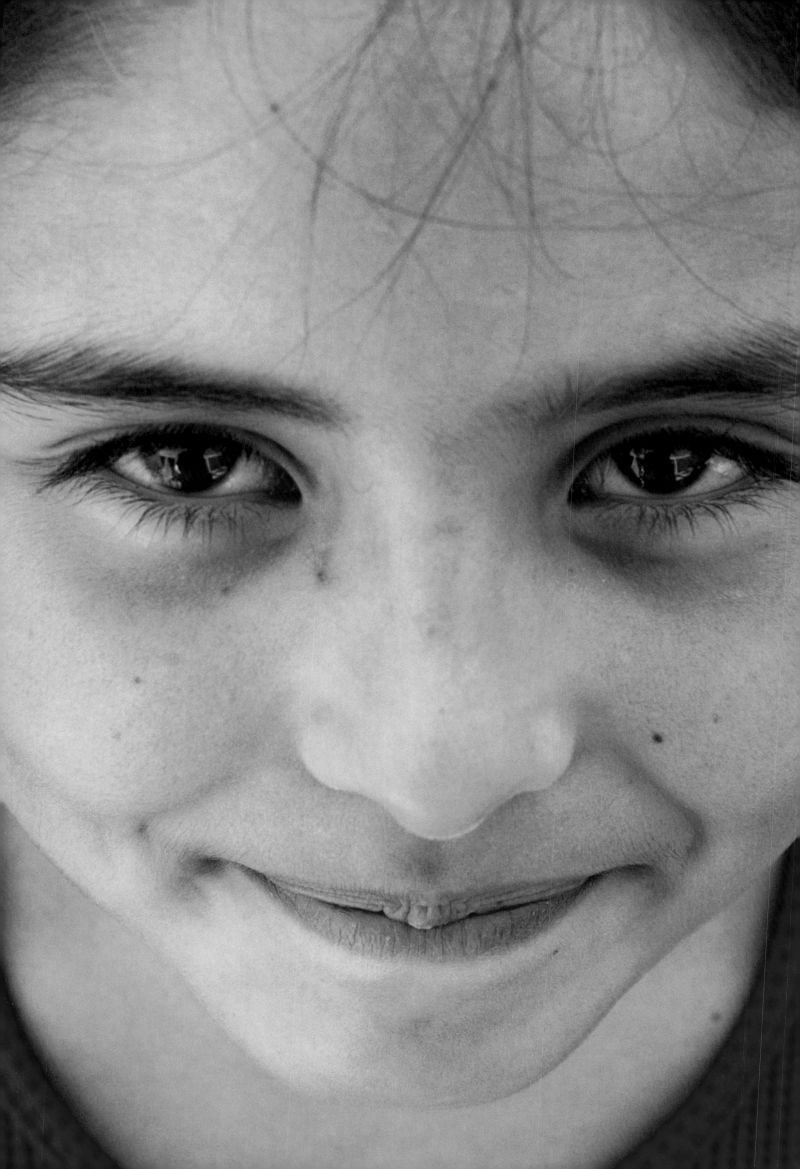

Clare, Daniel, Erik & Kelly
Katja, Tamara & Sasha
Victor
Parojn
Natasha
Deeb
Happy
& Andrea

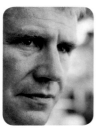

With this book, I would like to welcome you into the lives of 13 extraordinary young people.

They have one thing in common; they all have diabetes. Some of them were born with this lifelong chronic condition. A few of them had the ill fortune to live a lifestyle that prompted it. As individuals they are very different. They come from eight countries on four continents and represent different cultures, backgrounds and age groups. Some are battling ignorance and poverty; others have access to the most recent medical technology. So why is it that together their stories are interesting? And what is it that Novo Nordisk, as a world leader in diabetes care, hopes to achieve by telling their stories?

More than having diabetes in common, they have each found their own way to deal with a condition that never goes away. They refuse to let diabetes take over their lives, and they share a state of mind – a special place in their lives – where they find strength, optimism and renewed energy to fight their diabetes.

The ambition of this book has been to inspire the way we think about diabetes as a disease and people with diabetes as patients. By placing the individual before the disease, and by going behind their disease stories and into their real stories, as we have done in this book, we believe that we have an opportunity to help people

with diabetes find their own personal reserves to live a full life with – and despite of – their diabetes. We have chosen to look at diabetes through the fresh eyes of children and young people because through their eyes we can see, understand and ultimately impact the future of diabetes – their future. We hope that it can inspire people across all age groups.

At Novo Nordisk we have a stated ambition to lead the fight against diabetes and ultimately defeat diabetes. This book is an invitation to people with diabetes, their families, healthcare professionals and health policy-makers, who share our desire to change the way we think about and approach diabetes, to work with us to build a better future in diabetes care. The proceeds from the sales of this book will go towards helping children with special needs to live a full life with diabetes. Children like Happy from Tanzania, whose story is in this book.

Lastly, a heartfelt thank you to all the people behind these eight stories; the children, young adults and their parents, for inviting us into their private lives and giving us all a better understanding of how they cope with their diabetes. By telling your stories you have made an important contribution to improving the future of diabetes care.

Lars R. Sørensen

Lars Rebien Sørensen
President and CEO, Novo Nordisk

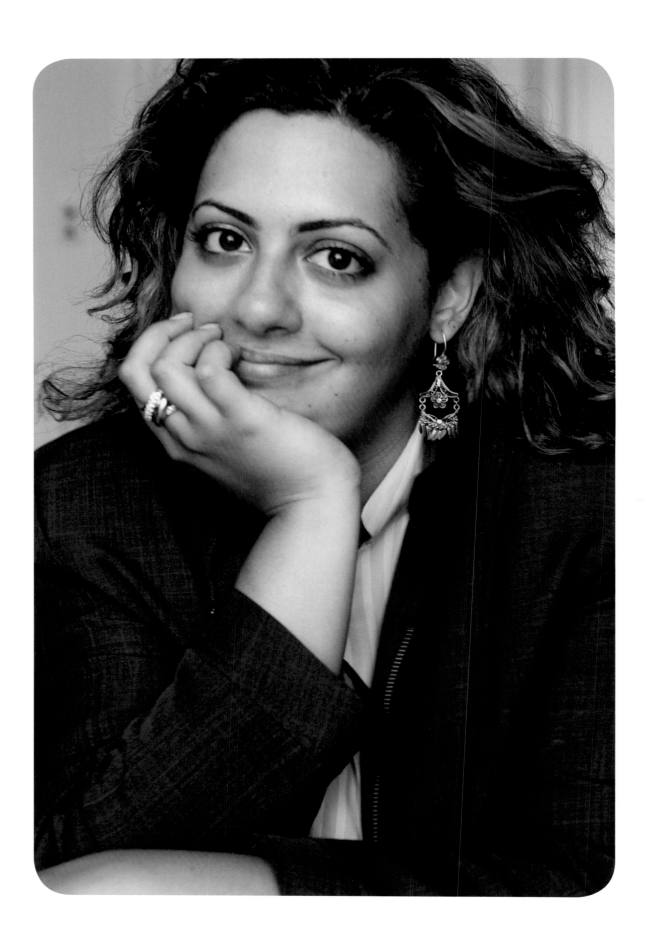

8 stories – 13 persons out of 177 million...

A little over a year ago, I had no real understanding of what diabetes truly was. To me, a person with diabetes simply had to refrain from including too much sugar in his or her diet. I knew nothing of a diabetes prevalence around the world, or of the role one's lifestyle plays in increasing the risk of a diagnosis of diabetes. I never knew that I *myself* could be at risk. I began to care; not only about diabetes and people diagnosed with diabetes, but also about an entire world out there that knows nothing about diabetes and what it could mean to their lives.

Suddenly, I found myself on a whirlwind of a journey, travelling the world and listening to stories of incredible people and their lives with diabetes.

USA, RUSSSIA, DENMARK, THAILAND, UK, JORDAN, TANZANIA & MEXICO.

Deeb, Victor, Clare, Daniel, Erik, Kelly, Parojn, Andrea, Happy, Natasha, Katja, Sasha and Tamara all told me about diabetes; about what it means to live with it.

I learned about the importance of having a strong character, the dedication and willpower and commitment to persevere. I saw how people all over the world are not only different in their cultures and ways of living, but also in the way they live with their diabetes. And I also saw how we are all the same.

We all want to live full lives, without the worry of pain and disease. We want to share our happy moments with loved ones and work hard at fulfilling all of our dreams. We want to learn from our mistakes and help others benefit from our experiences. I saw these desires in these young people, and I can never thank them enough for opening my eyes.

The purpose of this book is to open all of our eyes and introduce us to the extraordinary people out there for whom Novo Nordisk truly works. I have been inspired by each and every one of the stories I have been told, and I hope that I, in turn, will inspire you with the telling of each story. I hope you will see the strength in each of these incredible people, and I hope you will also learn from their experiences, as I did.

The stories in this book show how each of the remarkable individuals I met are learning to live with diabetes. They share their stories for one reason and one reason only: they want to raise awareness throughout the world of what living with diabetes is really like, because only awareness generates the power to create change.

Hala Khalaf

Author

Clare, Daniel, Erik & Kelly

These young adults, at various stages of living with diabetes, share a common belief:

life is so much more, so much bigger and better than diabetes.

Katja, Tamara & Sasha

The girls, brought together by diabetes, are comforted in the knowledge there is always someone

out there who understands, and who can be trusted.

Victor

Victor, a 10-year-old boy with type 1 diabetes, and his mother, Merete, are role models for

every person who finds himself or herself in their situation.

Parojn

Each individual living with diabetes deals with this difficult situation in his or her own

unique way.

Natasha

Gradually, she uncovers a well of self-confidence and strength gurgling deep within her.

She no longer wants to miss out on life. She wants to fight her diabetes and live.

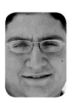

Deeb

Deep down inside, beneath the feelings of fulfilment, serenity and hope that surge through

prayer, Deeb knows that the necessary transformation can only come from within him.

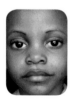

Happy

After eating, the quiet, inactive and withdrawn girl that was Happy miraculously becomes a vivacious,

chattering and lively child. Happy's parents cannot afford wholesome meals or regular snacks for their

growing daughter.

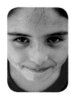

Andrea

Andrea knows that by taking care of herself, she can live her life, with all it has to offer, and

she does not want to waste a minute missing out on the beauty of living.

Table of Contents

Clare, Daniel, Erik & Kelly

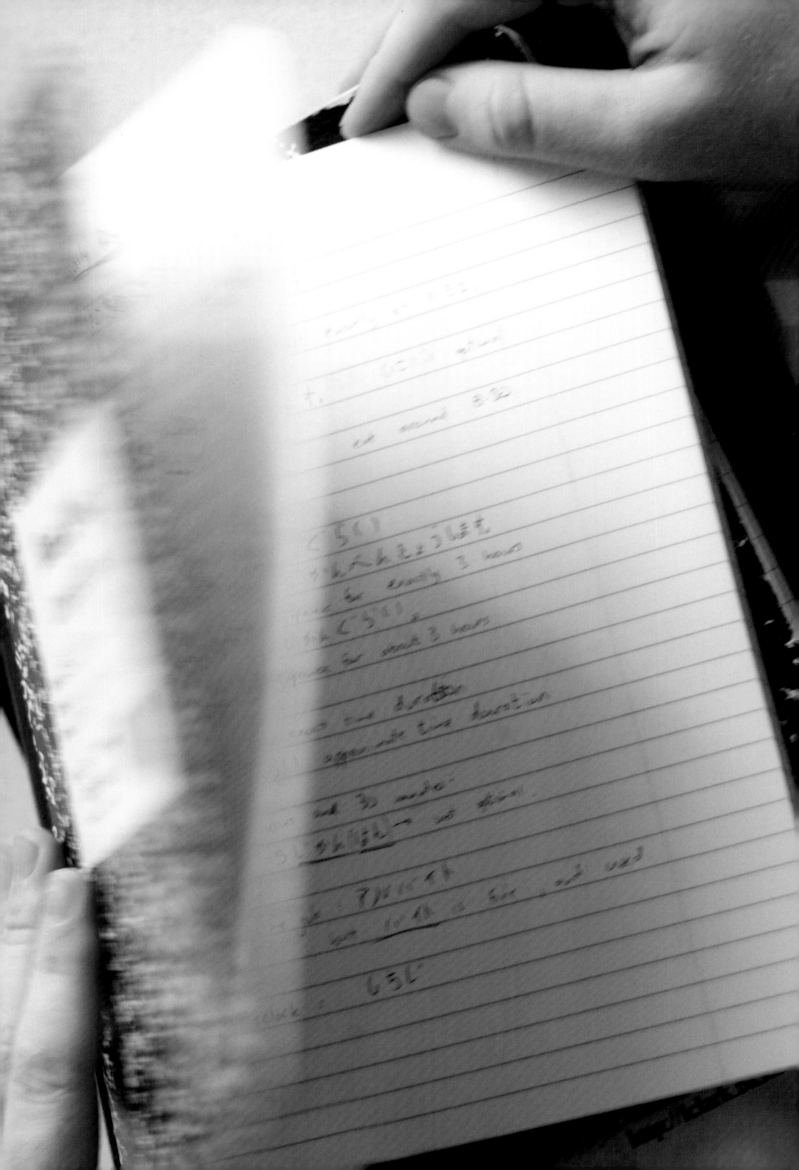

Clare Rosenfeld, Daniel Tolle, Erik Dunham & Kelly Hansen

What spirit! What intelligence! What awareness! Spending time with Clare, Daniel, Erik and Kelly is a pleasure. These young adults, at various stages of living with diabetes, share a common belief: life is so much more, so much bigger and better than diabetes. Their maturity is astonishing, and there is a lot to learn from them.

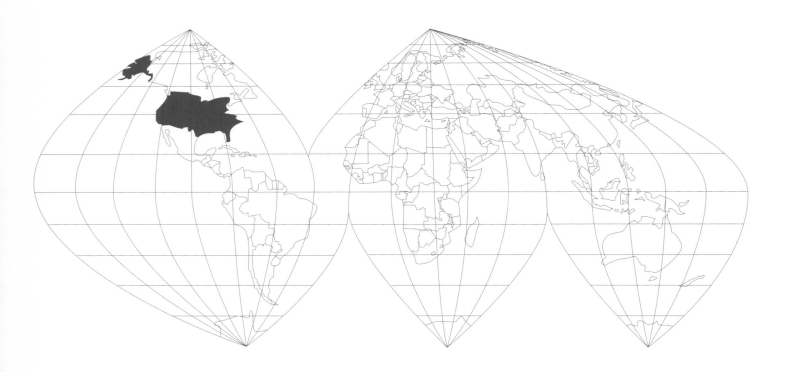

USA

The USA in North America comprises 48 contiguous states bounded by Canada, Mexico, Alaska and Hawaii. The populous eastern states are bordered by the Atlantic Ocean in the north and the Gulf of Mexico in the south. The central states form a vast interior plain, drained by the Mississippi-Missouri river system. The Rocky Mountains on the east and the Pacific Margin on the west are separated by a system of intermontane plateaus and basins.

The USA has abundant natural resources: coal, petroleum, natural gas and minerals as well as forests and agriculture. Although it is the largest energy consumer, the USA must still import vast quantities of energy resources. Manufacturing is diverse. The main products are: Iron, steel, aluminium metals and products, machinery, transport equipment (motor vehicles and aircraft), electrical and electronic goods, food products, chemicals, textiles and clothing. The USA has the largest economy in the world, based mainly on manufacturing and services, including banking and finance.[1]

STATUS Republic
POPULATION 295,734,134 [2]
PEOPLE WITH DIABETES 18,200,000 [3]
LANGUAGES English, Spanish, Amerindian languages
RELIGIONS Protestant, Roman Catholic, Sunni Muslim, Jewish, Mormon

Portland, OREGON
STATUS State
POPULATION 3,750,000

[1] The country information is summarized from The Times Atlas of the World - Consice Edition, 1996.

[2] U.S. Census Bureau, International Data Base, September 30, 2004.

[3] American Diabetes Association Web site, 2002 www.diabetes.org

"When we're all together, we're all *normal*!"

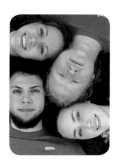

The four jostle one another in the cafeteria as they wait for their deli sandwiches. Their hectic class schedule does not allow them to get together to share a meal very often, so they are making the most out of the time they have, sharing stories and jokes.

Carrying their trays of food, the four students settle into a booth. Erik takes a bite out of his sandwich, but Clare, Daniel and Kelly bring out their glucometers first.

"I call Erik the 'fake diabetic,'" says Dan with a chuckle, as he waits for his glucometer to give him a reading on his blood sugar level.

Clare and Kelly smile and shake their heads at Dan's humour, while they wait for their own readings to register. A friendly competition has sprung up between the girls and Dan; whoever has the most ideal blood sugar reading gets a loud cheer. Dan wins the day's test and he bites into his sandwich with satisfaction while the two girls adjust their pumps to give them more insulin.

Erik observes the others as he takes a drink from his small milk carton. He had already taken his pill for the day and does not have to concern himself with insulin injections. And he does not mind being labelled the 'fake diabetic.'

He knows his type 2 diabetes is different from the type 1 diabetes of the other three. But regardless, he feels a connection with them; it is a connection all four share.

"Hanging out with the other three, I just feel great," says Kelly. "It's so cool to have fun with people who completely understand your situation. And when we're all together, we're all *normal*! Anyone who *doesn't* have diabetes is the odd one out!"

DIFFERENT BUT THE SAME

Clare Rosenfeld, Daniel Tolle, Erik Dunham and Kelly Hansen are all students at the Lewis and Clark College in Portland, Oregon. The four, alike in so many ways, have one fundamental thing in common: they all have diabetes.

Their stories, however, have different twists and turns. Clare and Dan, who both have type 1 diabetes, have known each other for years, and were diagnosed, respectively, at the ages seven and six.

Kelly, who also has type 1 diabetes, was diagnosed three years ago when she was 16. Although she says she has forgotten what life was like before her diabetes, she is still struggling to adjust.

Erik, on the other hand, has type 2 diabetes, and only learned of the fact a year ago on his 19th birthday. He sees diabetes as the best thing that could ever have

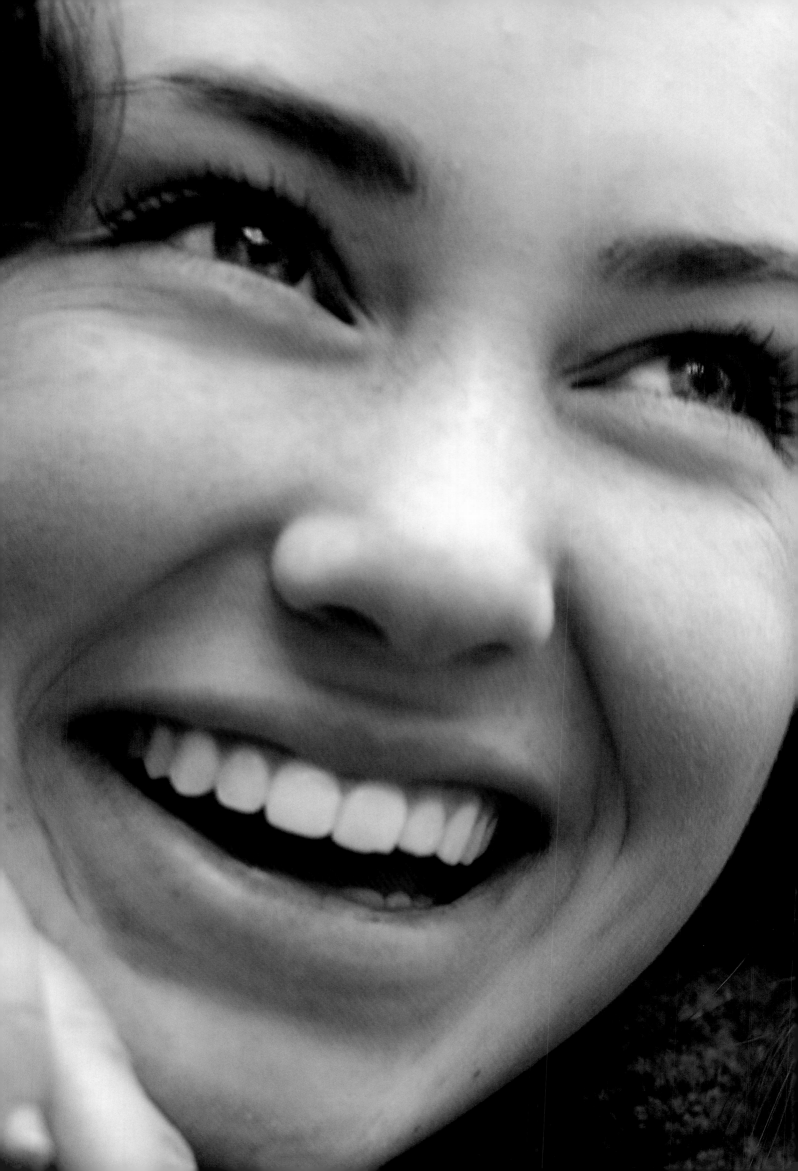

happened to him and he works hard at mastering and controlling his disease.

Each one of the four students lives with his or her diabetes in a completely different manner: their choices are personal and individual. Clare uses advocacy and a dedication to raise awareness to fight back, choosing to take action and help others learn from her own experiences. Dan's humour and laughter mask a deep commitment to do the best he can, and he relies heavily on his work as a diabetes camp counsellor to provide him with the necessary support to live with his diabetes. Erik's analytical personality has helped him reach the conclusion that his diabetes is a simple and straightforward problem than can be dealt with efficiently; he has created a process for himself that is working. Kelly, too, has identified a formula that works for her; she must make diabetes fit her lifestyle and her struggle is slowly beginning to ease.

Having found one another, the four rely on their friendship to help them cope. Their problems are reflected in each other and that bond makes them stronger. They have their bad days when they battle moments of frustration and anger. And yet, they all possess the strong mindset that allows them to battle against giving in to diabetes. They are living lives that are full and varied and together they have reached a common conclusion: they are normal.

CLARE:
///I know I can make a difference."

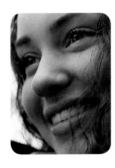

Clare is the youngest of the four – she is 18-years-old and in her freshman year of college. She is working towards a double major in chemistry and international affairs, and the young woman is focused and aware of what she wants.

"I love educating people about diabetes," she says, her face becoming instantly animated as she describes her passion. "I was diagnosed when I was seven and I gave my first speech about diabetes and what it's like to live with it three months later."

Clare's parents had gone away on a brief vacation, leaving Clare and her younger sister, Jenna, with an aunt and uncle. "My aunt and uncle took me and Jenna and all of the cousins to a summer fair one afternoon and I was drinking a *lot* of water! I had a huge sugary drink, then finished my sister's drink, then collapsed on a bench and complained of a headache and of feeling terrible." Clare's aunt, who is a retired nurse, recognised her niece's symptoms, and advised Clare's parents to take her to the hospital immediately.

"I found myself in the hospital for an entire week and then they told me that I had diabetes – a disease – and my first thought was, 'Oh my God, I'm going to die,'" says Clare, laughing at her initial reaction. But, for a seven-year-old, the experience was very frightening and Clare still remembers how scared she was. "I remember my mother asking if I would get over it!"

The little girl had heard rumours that she could not eat sugar any longer and panicked, thinking that cotton candy would be off limits forever. "I remember crying a lot. It was a difficult time."

However, Clare and her parents don't let much get them down. On their way home from the hospital, after stopping at a local pharmacy for insulin and other diabetes supplies that Clare might need, the family drove to the office of the American Diabetes Association (ADA) in their city of Eugene, Oregon. There, they signed themselves up for education courses on diabetes.

"The ADA hooked us up with another family that had a little girl, Anne, who also had diabetes, and I will never forget her. It was at that moment I realised how important it was to have support available from other people with diabetes – and to realise you are not alone."

That moment, coupled with something Clare's mother, Kari, had told her, made all the difference in Clare's approach to diabetes from that day onwards. When her feelings of anger threatened to overwhelm her, Clare turned to her mother.

"My mom said to me, 'Clare, you can be angry about diabetes; that's okay. But don't take that anger out on yourself. Take that passion and that energy and do something good with it. Accomplish something, instead of being destructive towards yourself."

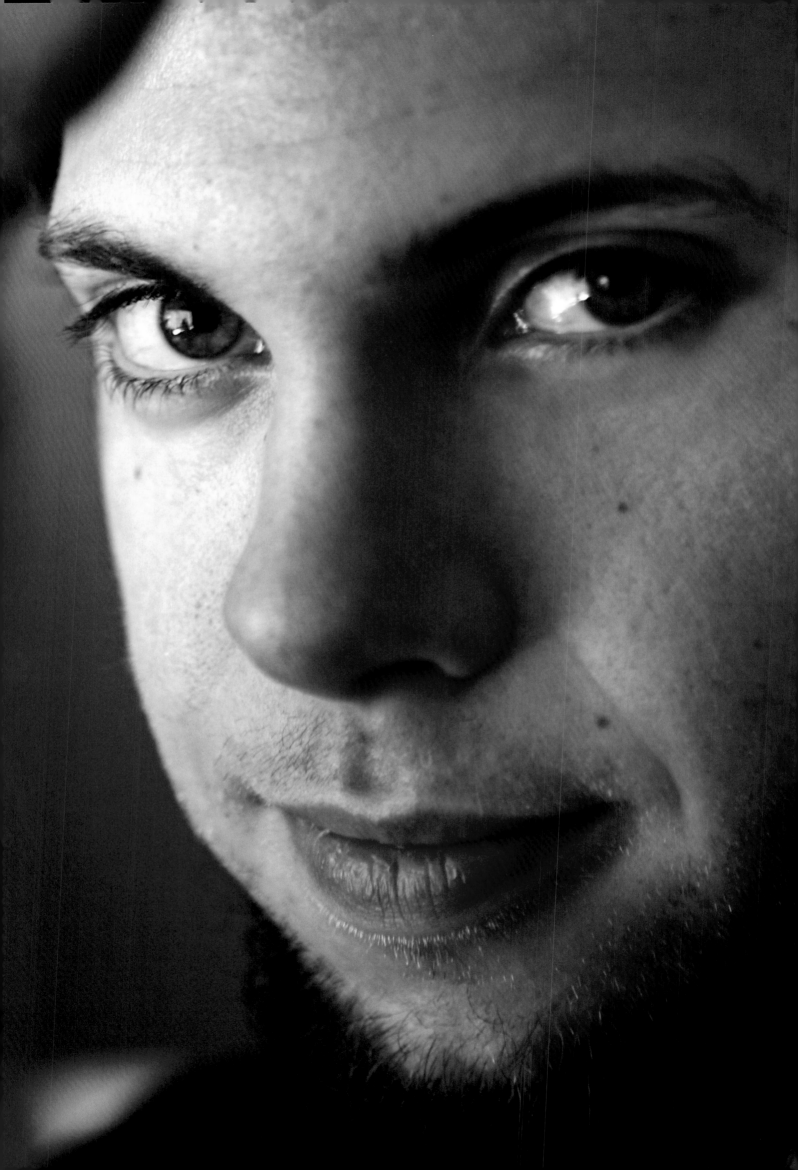

Clare did just that. Supported by her mother, she began educating herself on diabetes to gain control and power over the disease. By educating herself, she acquired the ability to educate others and found ways of helping them – just as Anne had helped her.

From that moment, more than 11 years ago, until today, Clare has worked tirelessly to raise awareness of diabetes, not only in the United States but also throughout the world. She is an International Diabetes Youth Ambassador and takes her work very seriously.

"It is so important to have support from peers who understand what you are going through and I want to give that support to others. At the same time, it is also important to be well-educated in diabetes – and to understand what diabetes really is," she stresses. "If you educate one person about diabetes, then you have really educated twenty others, because people pass their knowledge along."

Clare feels that it is her advocacy work and her desire to help others that has helped her to deal with her own diabetes. "Being a peer mentor for other people and giving them the support they need taught me how to support myself. You only become master of yourself when you have to be strong for other people."

She flips her long, curly, brown hair over her shoulder and relaxes slightly.

"I don't mean to sound so intense. I like to let loose and have a good time as well!" She laughs at herself, describing her interest in books, writing poetry, taking dance lessons with her boyfriend and scuba diving.

Clare obtained her scuba diving certification just a few days after her 12th birthday to become, as far as she knows, the youngest certified scuba diver with diabetes.

"Diabetes cannot stop you from accomplishing anything. In fact, diabetes has added to my life and given me an entirely new perspective. I want a cure more than anything, but the truth is, if I could go back in time and have a choice of life with or without diabetes, I would choose to live with it. I have become a stronger person because of diabetes."

DANIEL:

❚❚ Can't do it without friends and diabetes camp."

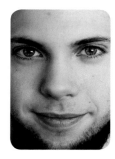

Daniel, with his piercing blue eyes, dyed black hair and curly brown beard, loves to laugh and likes it best when everyone around him is also laughing. "I like humour," he says. "I think humour is really important. It makes everything in the world just so much better."

The 20-year-old grew up in Portland and is currently in his sophomore year of college. He wants to become a research scientist and is considering a double major in chemistry and biology. Dan was diagnosed with type 1 diabetes when he was six-years-old.

"Just before I was diagnosed, my dad and I were travelling by car from Chicago to Portland, which is a pretty long drive. My dad told me about how he had to stop, like every hour or so, for me to go to the bathroom and get a drink of water." Dan's father did not recognise the symptoms, but his mother, who is an internal medicine doctor, rushed Dan off to get a urine sample analysis.

"I was so young and at that age, you don't really grasp the concept of 'You're going to have this thing forever and it's supposed to be a bad thing,'" says Dan. "So I was pretty good about it. I never put up a fuss."

However, many years later, when Dan finally found himself alone on a college campus, he decided to see how far he could stretch the rules.

"I thought to myself, 'Well, do I *really* have to take my insulin shot at every meal?'" He pans for effect to an invisible audience and flashes a grin. "It's a terrible idea, *terrible* idea to skip your insulin shot – take it from me!"

"You get *so* sick and you feel *so* crappy and then you go back to taking your shots when you have to, and you think, 'This is great! Why was I so stupid before? What was I thinking?'"

Dan knows he is never alone and has never had the

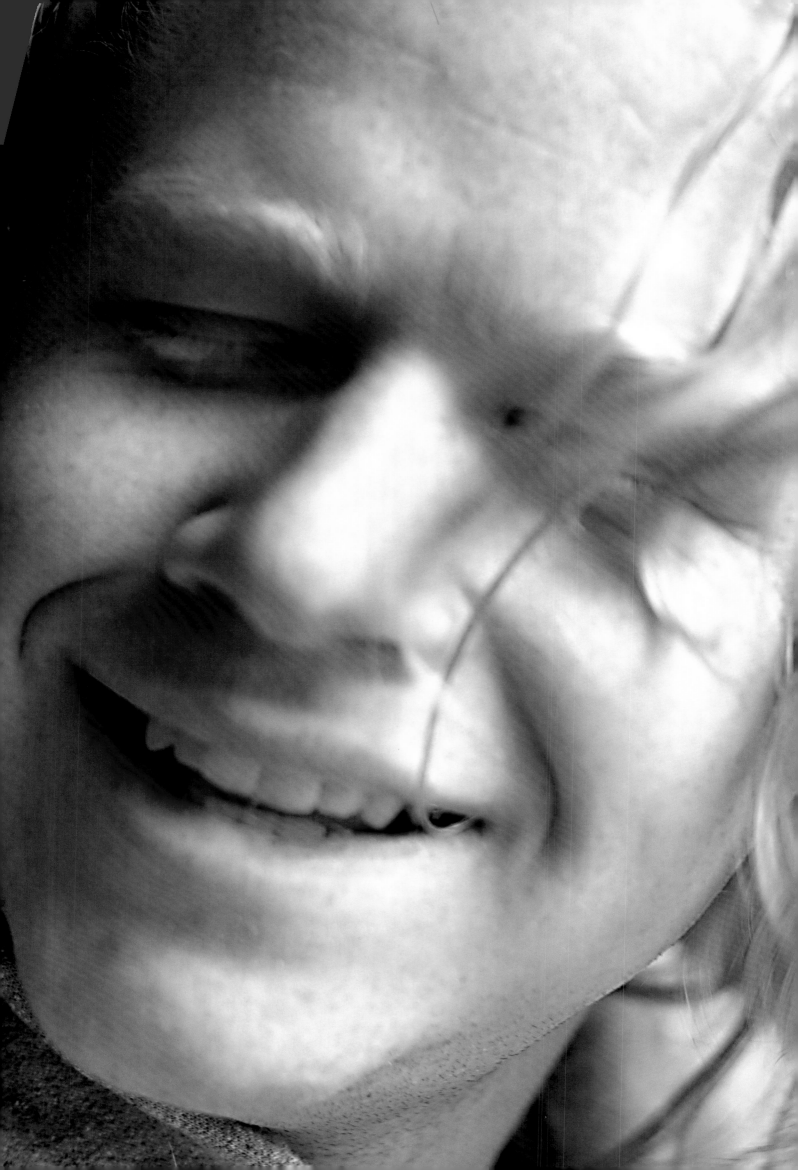

reason to feel as if he was. Part of that is thanks to the many experiences he has had at diabetes camp.

"I love camp. Camp changed my life. I don't know *what* I would do if I couldn't go to camp still," he says. The ADA organises camps all over the United States that cater for children with diabetes, and Dan has spent his summers at such camps every year since his diagnosis. For the past two summers, he has worked as a camp counsellor at his childhood diabetes camp. He says the experiences have been the most rewarding of his life.

In camp, the children learn the practicalities of life with diabetes – including how to test their blood sugar, how to give themselves insulin shots, and so on. And, like Daniel, they learn the value of long-term management and the importance of gaining independence. "I had such a positive experience at camp, and I really want to allow the kids that continue to come there to have that also. I remember how important it was for me and I want to ensure that it's still available.

"Camp is one of the most important things in my life. I doubt I would have done remotely as well diabetes-wise and health-wise without camp. I probably would not have learned to do my own shots for several more years, nor been so consistent with testing my blood sugar. I wouldn't have been updated on the most recent medical technology. And, I wouldn't have met Clare!"

For Dan, the friends that understand his diabetes are essential. Friends like Clare, Kelly and Erik are people he can count on. Whether he needs someone to talk to, hug, or beg strips from, he knows he can go to them, and that they will be there for him.

ERIK:
❚❚There are many worse things that can happen."

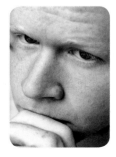

Erik's doctors admitted to being baffled by the 20-year-old's diagnosis of type 2 diabetes. Erik, who had just turned 19 at the time, is healthy, physically active and at an ideal weight. There is some family history of diabetes, but that is all.

"I am not going to waste my time wondering why," says Erik, his tone firm and determined. "I figured, 'It's just life. So deal with it.'"

Erik grew up in Kennewick, a town in the rural southeast area of Washington State. Like Dan, Erik is in his sophomore year of college, and is double majoring in mathematics and German studies.

"I love sports. I've always played many different kinds of sports – football and basketball, ultimate Frisbee and running – and I wanted to play tennis for the college team," he says. Tennis at Lewis and Clark College falls under the jurisdiction of the National Collegiate of Athletic Associations (NCAA).

"Because tennis is an NCAA sport, I had to undergo a physical." Erik needed his doctor to clear him medically, so that he could join the team. However, his physical uncovered high blood sugar levels, and before long he was diagnosed with type 2 diabetes.

"There were all sorts of things I didn't know then, and really, I'm still learning about everything, but mostly," says Erik, "I didn't know how rare it is for someone like me to have type 2 diabetes."

Erik's diagnosis had little effect on him. There is nothing about his diabetes that makes him feel sick. As a result, he does not feel that it altered his life dramatically.

"All I have to do is continue to exercise regularly and to eat right – and, of course, take my pills. But that's it for me. It's so easy. I just don't see the big deal."

Erik's analytical attitude has driven him to conclude that many worse things could have happened to him and, in fact, diabetes is a very *good* thing to have happened to him.

"I am more aware of my body than any kid my age," he says. "Diabetes forces me to be healthier than I ever was before. I help myself by fighting it, and I reap the benefits."

Erik enjoys a good challenge. For example, he has a pas-

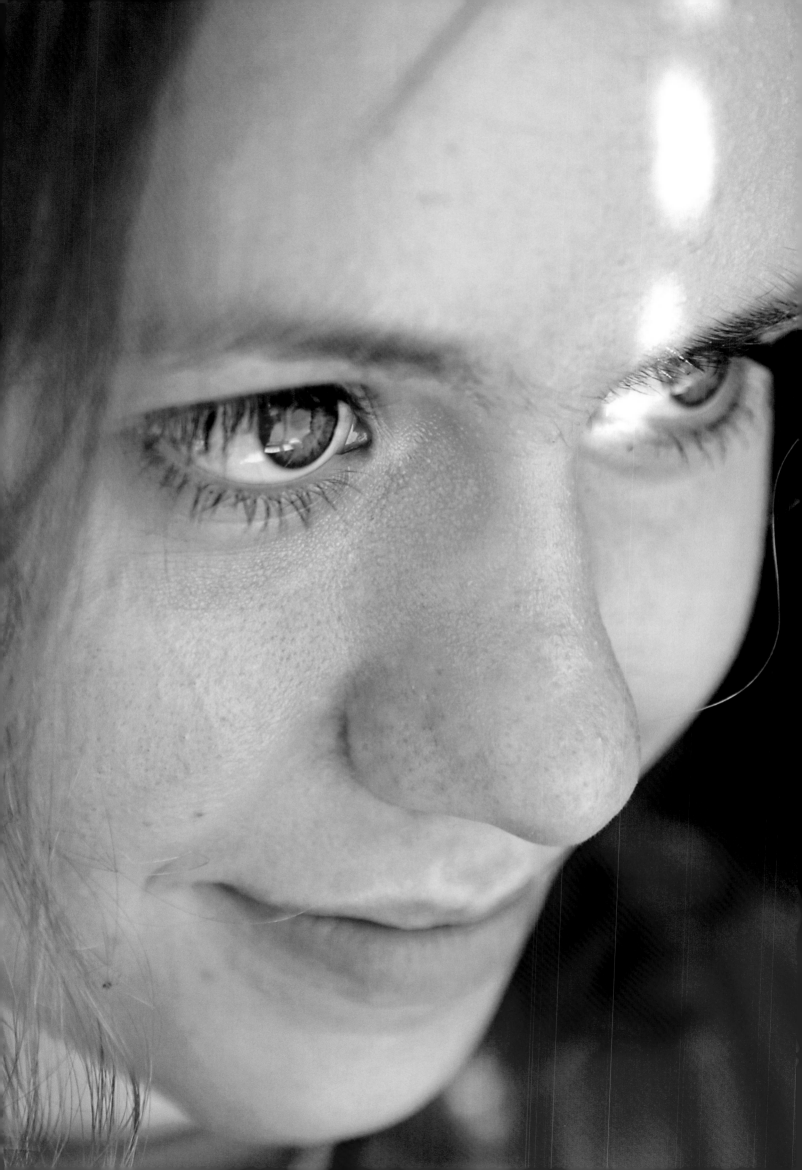

sion for solving Rubik cubes. To him, challenges present the idea of self-mastery and that is how he views his diabetes.

"I want to be in control of myself and not a victim of myself," he states. His fascination with mathematics and languages stems from that belief since both interests involve problem solving. To him, mathematics and languages are codes to be cracked.

"I'm not good at just learning information. I like to figure things out," he explains. "And with diabetes, I've figured out what I need to do – and I just do it," he says, running his hands through his Viking-like blonde hair.

Erik realises that he has the option of ignoring his diabetes and not taking care of himself. But that's not an option he exercises.

"Why would I hurt myself intentionally? I have the ability to control and to fight, so why wouldn't I? I am not going to go down because of some disease that is so easy for me to handle. That's how I look at it."

Diabetes holds no embarrassment for Erik. What would be embarrassing would be to allow diabetes to defeat him. That is why, he explains, he refuses to lose his self-respect by allowing a disease that can be self-managed to control him.

"People deal with so much worse! I don't mean to be dismissive, but I have the ability to deal with this problem and get rid of it as a problem, so that's what I do," says Erik, who wants to learn even more about diabetes and the pandemic that type 2 is becoming around the world. He truly believes that when much is given to an individual, then much is expected *from* that individual. He has been given all he needs to deal with his disease, and so he, in turn, wants to make a difference.

"I want to give back. I have had everything I need all my life and I am from a small percentage of people in the world who can say that. I feel obligated to make an impact. I want to do something with my life. Maybe my diabetes will help me achieve that."

KELLY:

▮▮It's a balancing act that you have to adapt to."

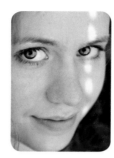

Kelly recently turned 19 and on Valentine's Day will celebrate her third anniversary of being diagnosed with type 1 diabetes. Before moving to Oregon for her college education, she lived in Alaska. At Lewis and Clark, Kelly is pursuing a double major in biology and music education.

"Actually, I'm thinking of dropping the music education to concentrate more on history," she says, gesturing towards the pictures of mummies, tombs and pyramids on the walls of her room. "I have a fetish for Egyptology! I am just interested in so many different things. I can't make up my mind on what I want to concentrate on since I want to do everything!" Kelly's blue-green eyes sparkle and she fingers the Egyptian cartouche she always wears around her neck. She loves to travel, and dreams of the moment she finds herself in Egypt.

For six months before her diagnosis, Kelly had been feeling extremely fatigued. She was drinking at least three bottles of water per class in high school, and losing weight unintentionally. "I remember walking through a grocery store with my mom and seeing these gallons of apple juice and thinking, 'Oh! I could drink that right now! All of it, all of it!'" she says, laughing at the memory.

Eventually, Kelly sought a medical opinion, and she was diagnosed with type 1 diabetes. She stayed at the hospital for four days, trying to come to terms with the new addition to her life.

"I remember all the nurses saying, 'It's okay to be upset,' but I couldn't let myself be upset about it. I could see my parents were having a hard time and I thought that making a scene would upset them even more, so I didn't let myself show any feelings."

Soon, however, the knowledge that diabetes would be with her for the rest of her life got to Kelly. No matter how much she told herself that she could deal with it, she was terrified.

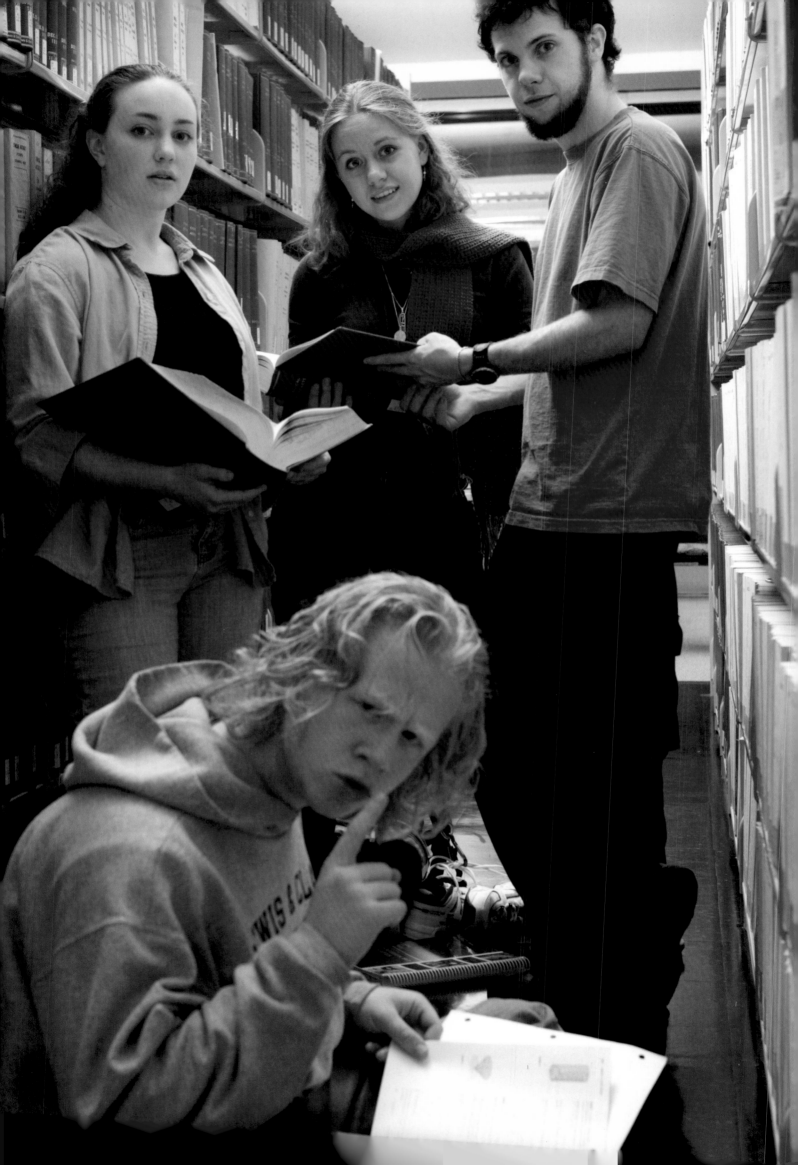

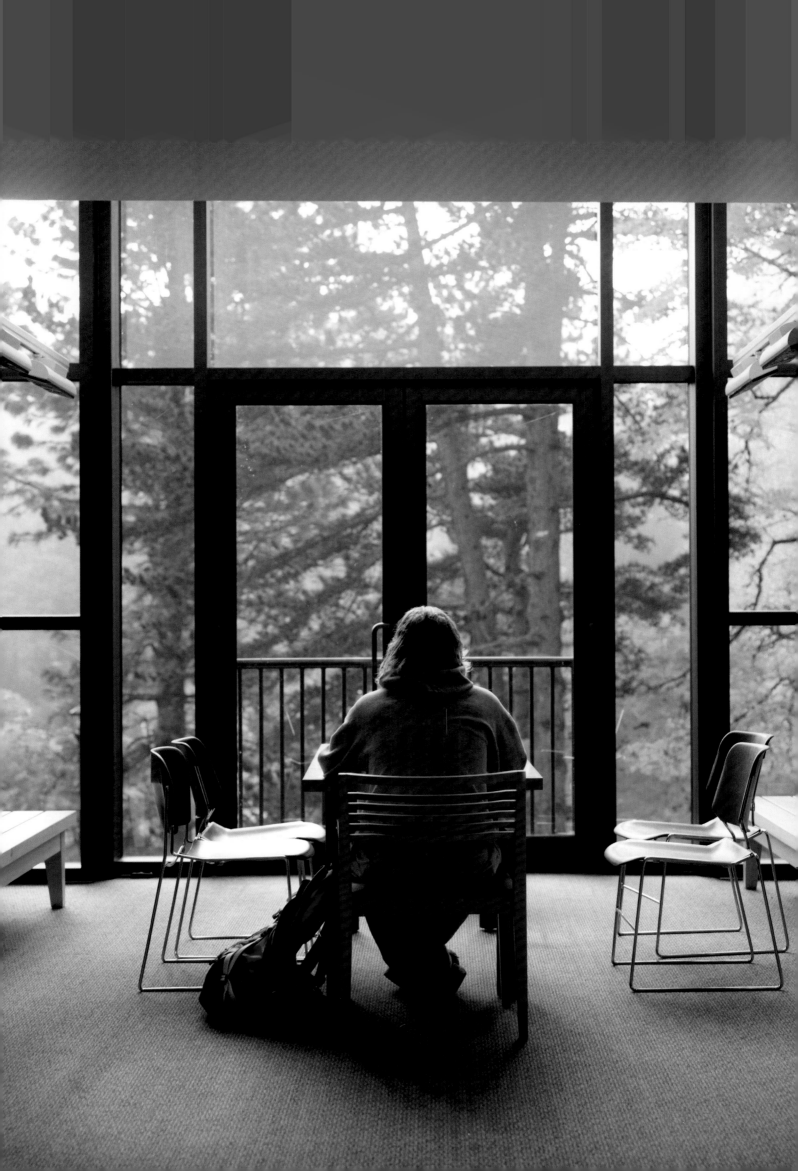

"I still get scared sometimes – I'm still learning all about this. I've figured out that diabetes is a balancing act. You have to figure out how to take care of yourself, but in the end, to make diabetes fit into your life. You have to adapt; you have to adapt to everything you do. Diabetes is just another new thing."

Kelly does not feel that she has adapted completely yet. Adjusting to the new experience of campus life makes regulating her blood sugar levels harder than it was before. She is very busy on campus, playing the French horn in the college orchestra and band in addition to attending classes and pursuing all her other interests like photography, French, reading and journal writing.

"It is unrealistic for me to say at this point that I am perfectly okay with having diabetes. It is difficult to have diabetes and to feel, somehow, that I am different from other people," says Kelly. She misses being able to eat anything she wants without having to think of the consequences. Plus, she worries about her blood sugar level. She also has to deal with having to count the number of carbohydrates a dish contains to determine how much insulin she needs.

"I just generally miss how carefree life without diabetes seemed. Every once in a while I get really frustrated," she admits. However, Kelly discovered that after the initial feelings of anger and depression, she found her own way to live with it and adjust it to fit into her life.

"For anyone who ends up in my shoes, know that diabetes is hard to deal with. But it is *never* worth it to give up." Kelly will do anything to make herself feel better during her moments of sadness, including using her music, art, pictures or books as a medium. She believes that the relationship growing between her, Clare, Dan and Erik will help her even further. Just knowing them, she says, is therapeutic.

For Kelly, being with Dan, Clare and Erik is "really cool." Like the others, she finds comfort in the knowledge that she is not the only one struggling with diabetes.

"There are other people out there who have this disease too, and are just as busy as I am, and they're fine and surviving."

The sense of normalcy she gets when she is with the others gives her the added confidence to go on. Kelly lives her life day to day, and works hard at not letting her diabetes get her down.

PEER SUPPORT

The four young adults want, more than anything, to raise awareness about their disease. They no longer want to be asked if diabetes is contagious, nor if it means they can never eat sugar.

They do not balk before the task of explaining their diabetes to curious friends. On the contrary, like Clare, they agree that the more people that know about diabetes, the better. However, they do appreciate the moments when they can sit back, lean against one another and not have to explain what "high" or "low" blood sugar means.

"It's nice to have a group like Dan and Clare and Erik, because I'm no longer the one that's different in my group of friends. Sometimes you need to hang out with other people who are like you," says Kelly.

Erik agrees. "It's neat to have a group of friends that can be so supportive and helpful and understanding," he says. "I didn't have that before, and I didn't know I wanted it."

Dan and Clare already know the value of understanding peers. Clare works tirelessly at providing that support to others worldwide, while Dan encourages the next generation of youth advocates at the local level through his counselling at diabetes camp.

For all four, diabetes has presented the biggest challenge thus far in their young lives. For some more than others, it has also presented obstacles to overcome. Most of all, however, diabetes has provided them with common pride. They are overcoming the challenge they face with positive attitude, perseverance, hard work and faith. They help one another and they wish to help others.

For Clare, Dan, Erik and Kelly – who now dub themselves 'the Fabulous Four' – their lives with diabetes are a cause for celebration.

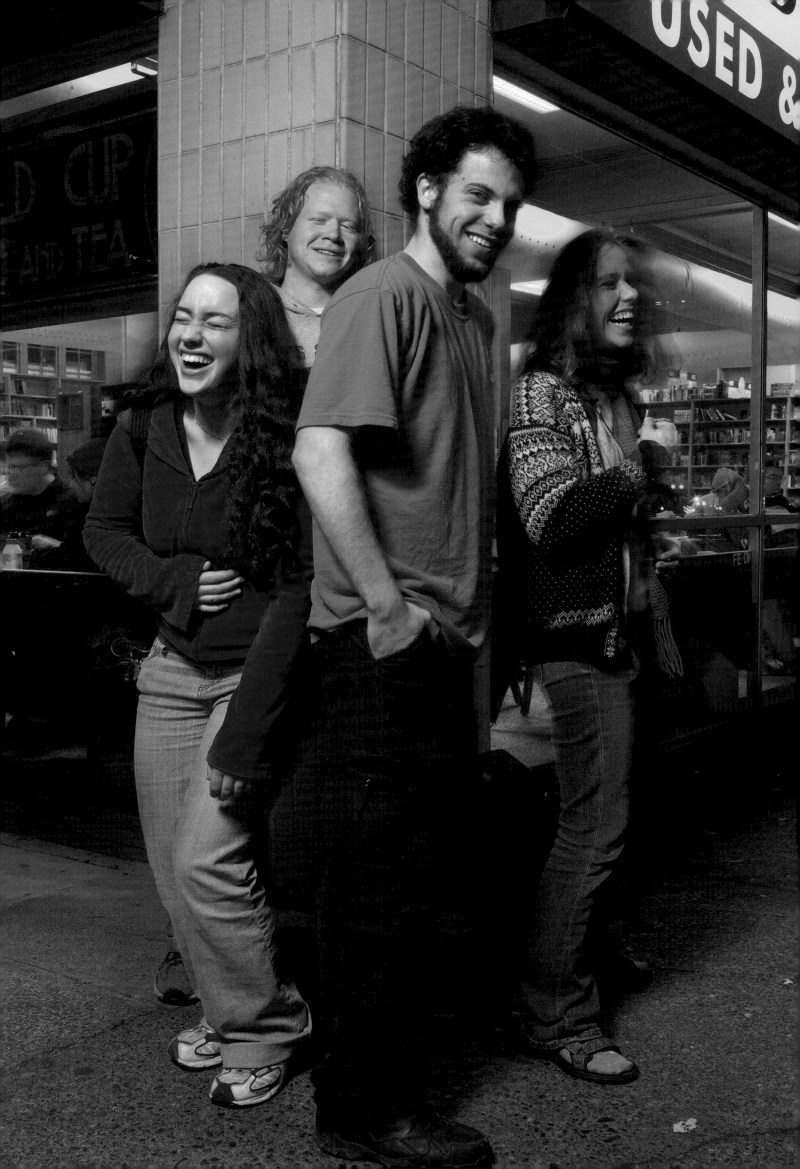

Katja, Tamara & Sasha

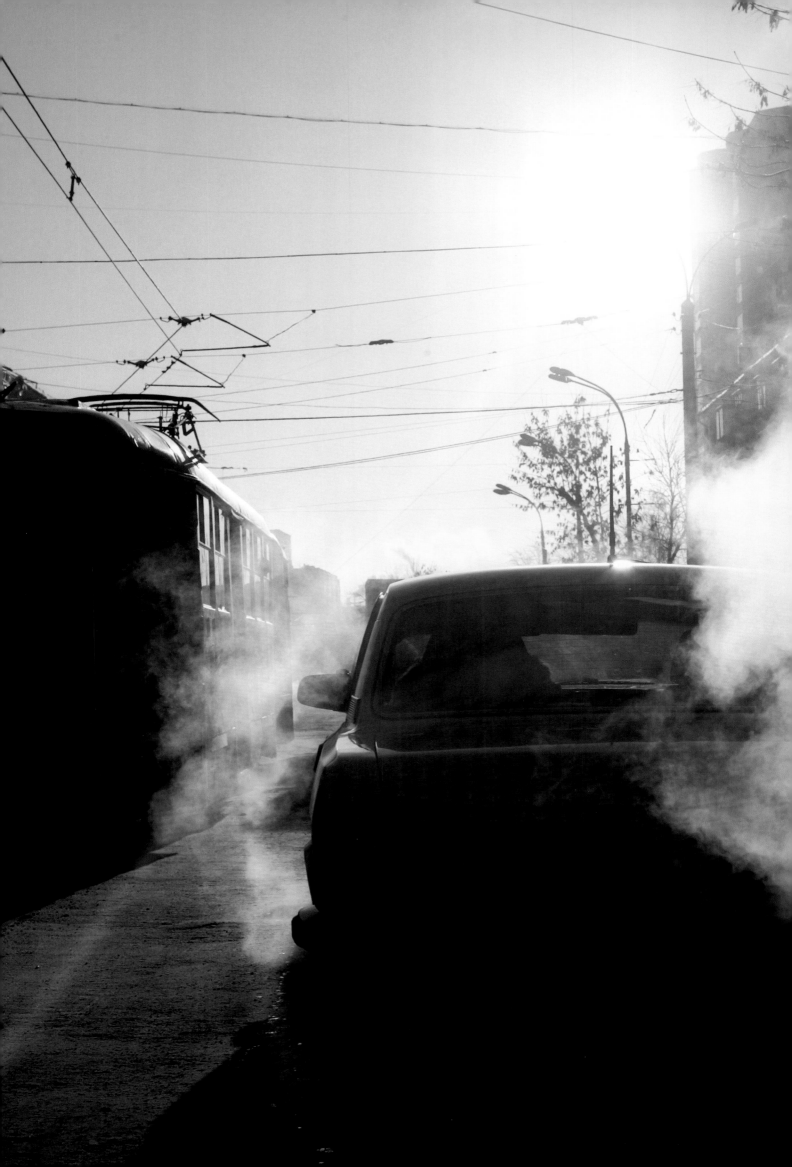

Katja Kornilova, Tamara Tutarauly & Sasha Koryako

A bitterly cold climate is characteristic of Pervouralsk, a small town near Russia's industrial city of Yekaterinburg. Yet the warm and loving nature of Katja, Tamara and Sasha overshadows the cold. The girls, brought together by diabetes, are comforted in the knowledge there is always someone out there who understands, and who can be trusted.

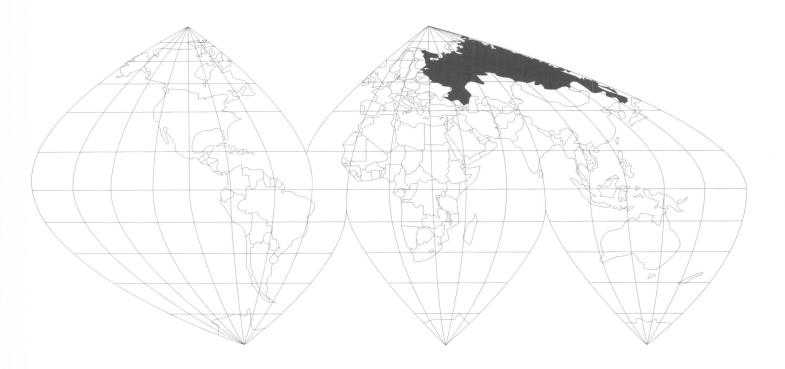

RUSSIA

The world's largest country covers northern Asia and the majority of eastern Europe. The climate is generally continental but with extreme temperatures that vary from arctic tundra to semi-arid steppe.

The Russian economy is based on heavy industry and raw materials such as petrol, natural gas, coal, asbestos, platinum, etc. Forests cover almost 40 per cent of Russia, and supply the important timber and pulp industry. Exports include mining, machinery, chemicals and textiles. Russia boasts one of the greatest fishing fleets in the world. However, the 1990s transition to a free market economy has led to rising unemployment.[1]

STATUS Republic
POPULATION 143,420,309 [2]
PEOPLE WITH DIABETES 9,700,000 [3]
LANGUAGES Russian, Tatar
RELIGIONS Russian Orthodox, Sunni Muslim, Jewish, Protestamt

[1] The country information is summarized from The Times Atlas of the World - Consice Edition, 1996.

[2] U.S. Census Bureau, International Data Base, September 30, 2004.

[3] International Diabetes Federation, 2004.

"Diabetes is our small world."

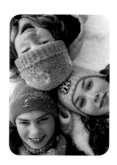

"Look at them. Aren't they pretty? They're brand new!" She shows off her silver bracelets and the other two girls nod appreciatively as they admire the accessories. The three of them huddle even closer together, their heads almost touching, as they giggle and laugh over the juicy bits they are whispering into one another's ears.

Their mothers draw their attention back to the menu and the three girls continue examining the many choices listed before them, unable to make up their minds as to what they would like to order. They ask each other's opinion on the various dishes and together use their fingers to count.

Yekaterina, Alexandra and Tamara are calculating approximately how many calories each dish they want to order contains. It is a complicated calculation, trying to figure out what they can have now by adding it to what they have already eaten earlier in the day.

All three girls have type 1 diabetes and counting calories is something they all got used to a long time ago.

"We go to diabetes school twice every year and there we learn lots of things, including how to count calories

and what to eat," says Yekaterina, better known as Katja to her family and friends.

"We didn't eat much today because we knew we would be going out to a restaurant and wanted to be sure we could have anything we wanted!" says Tamara, the youngest of the three girls.

"Besides, we all exercised today and had a nice, long walk and we can just adjust our dosage of insulin when we know how much we'll eat," says Alexandra, nicknamed Sasha, as she tilts her head to see how the light makes her bracelets shine.

After a few more minutes of negotiation, punctuated by regular sips of their apple juice, the three girls make up their minds. They all agree they must start with their favourite: 'Olivier' salad with veal tongue and roasted chicken breast. Katja chooses dumplings stuffed with three different kinds of meat for her main dish. Tamara claps her hands at the thought of a big plate of fried potatoes, mushrooms, onions and lard. Sasha settles for beef medallions with beans, pears and cranberry sauce.

All three are relieved to know that dishes of Russian specialties, featuring pickles, olives, white mushrooms and cured tomatoes with dill, are ordered for them to share. The girls place their dessert orders, their eyes shining at the thought of the pancakes and ice cream to come.

Having made their choices, the girls push their menus aside and huddle close together once again to pick up where they left off. Sasha's bracelets are inspected one more time and the girls all agree to give one another tastes from their different dishes.

Until the food arrives, they talk. After all, since they attend different schools, they have to catch up on a lot of gossip.

A CIRCLE OF TRUST

❙❙We have so much fun together that it's just a bonus for us that we have yet another thing in common, which happens to be diabetes. But it's not the only thing we have in common. It's a normal thing for us, so we don't really talk about it with each other."

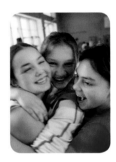

Katja Kornilova, Tamara Tutarauly and Sasha Koryako are three very different girls, brought together because they have something in common. The three girls, who all live in the town of Pervoularsk near the industrial city of Yekaterinburg in Russia, were diagnosed with type 1 diabetes at different stages in their lives.

Sasha has lived with diabetes for more than 10 years; she was diagnosed in 1994 at the age of four. Katja was diagnosed with diabetes in 1999 – just before her 11th birthday. Tamara has had the shortest experience with diabetes; she was diagnosed only three years ago, in August 2001.

The three are at various stages of living with their diabetes, but to all of them, diabetes is no big deal.

Katja, the oldest of the three and just a few months away from her 16th birthday, insists that the three never bring up the subject of diabetes when they are together.

"We have a lot of other interesting things to talk about. We can't waste what little time we have together talking about diabetes!" she exclaims.

Fifteen-year-old Sasha nods vigorously and nudges the other two girls, making them laugh.

"We talk about boys and music and clothes and movies and school. And boys!" All three erupt in giggles, falling against one another and clutching their sides.

When the laughter subsides and the three girls settle down, 13-year-old Tamara explains their outlook on diabetes even further.

"We have so much fun together that it's just a bonus for us that we have yet another thing in common, which happens to be diabetes. But it's not the only thing we have in common. It's a normal thing for us, so we don't really talk about it with each other."

However, behind their childlike banter and sunny smiles, the three girls admit to feeling a sense of peace whenever they are together, safe in the knowledge that they are not alone.

"When I am with the other girls," explains Sasha, "I feel safe and I feel like we have a special power together – that nothing can happen to us. We can take care of each other."

"I feel the same way," agrees Katja. "In comparison with people who don't have diabetes, I have more trust in these girls and I also have trust in myself when I am with them. We know what's right for us. Diabetes is our small world."

Perhaps because she is the youngest, Tamara is simply happy to know that there are other girls out there who also have diabetes and are nevertheless completely normal.

They are interested in the same things as Tamara. When she is with Katja and Sasha, Tamara feels she has every right to consider herself a normal teenager.

Nevertheless, the girls know that they are special in their own way – diabetes, after all, is not a trait they share with all their friends. Sometimes they worry what role diabetes may play in their future and fear losing their current control over the disease.

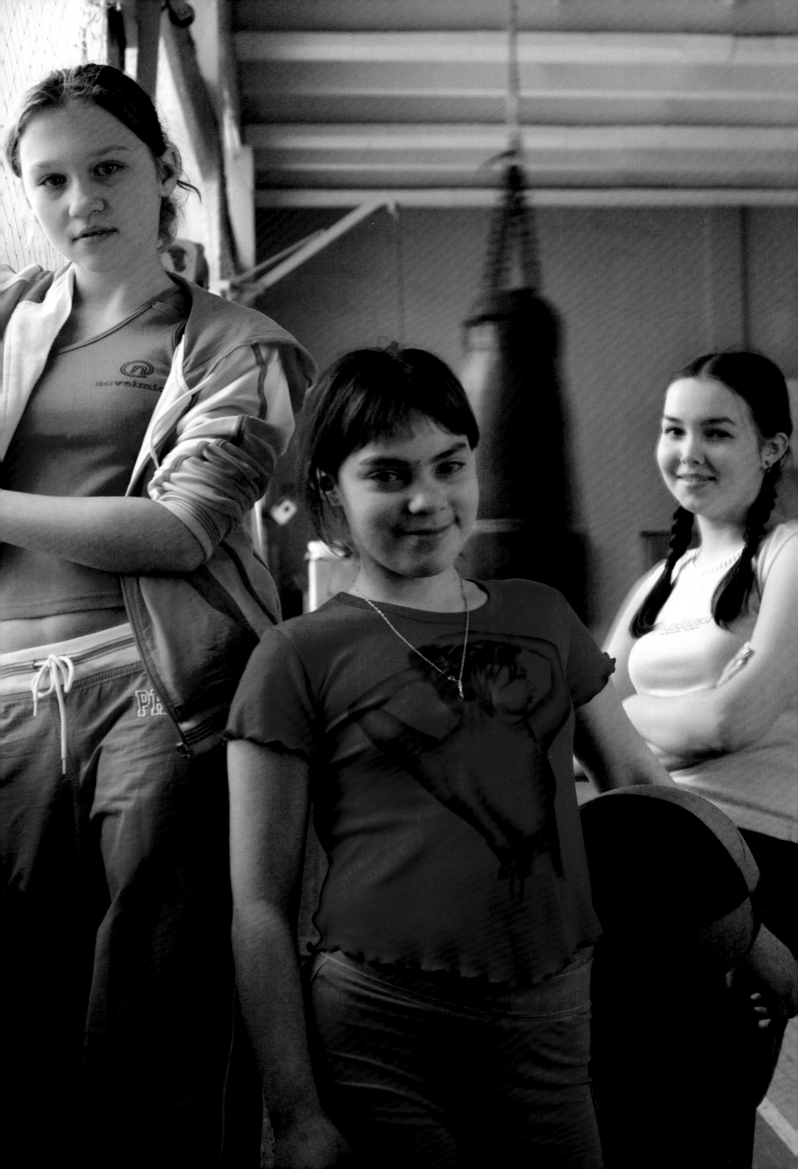

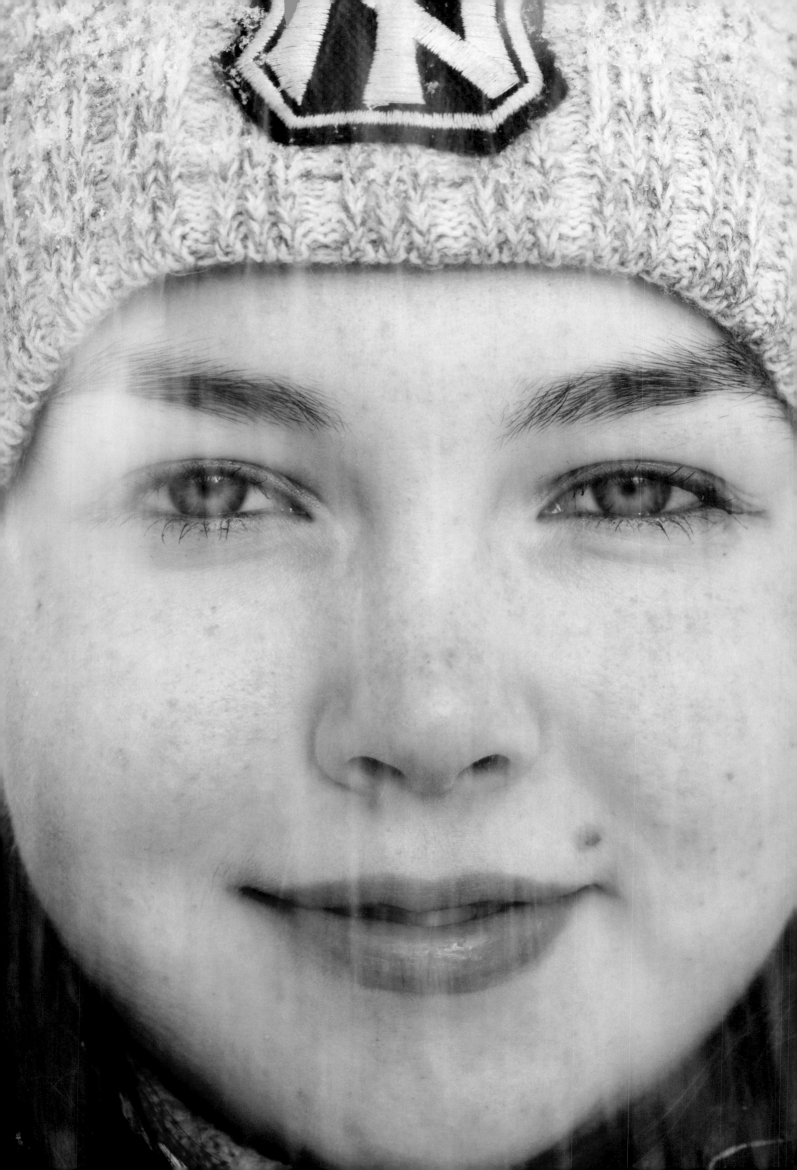

KATJA'S CHRONICLE

❚❚In Russia, sometimes people with diabetes are compared to drug addicts, because the addicts cannot live without their drugs and we cannot live without our insulin. But we are not addicts, we are normal. The addicts die from their drugs. But we survive and have better lives because of our insulin."

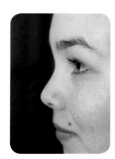 Katja, a mature teenager on the brink of becoming a young wo- man, has a poise not yet mastered by the other girls. She already knows the benefits of tossing her long, dark hair just so, and she loves outlining her slanted eyes with colourful eyeliner. Unlike the other girls, she already has a boyfriend, Tolya, a young man who has unwittingly wrapped himself around Katja's delicate little finger.

In February 1999, Katja and her best friend from child- hood decided to treat themselves to popsicles on their walk home from school. Soon after, both girls developed a throat infection, but Katja did not recover as quickly as her friend. Instead, she lost a considerable amount of weight and began drinking more water and other beverages than ever before.

Katja underwent some tests and the results showed she had type 1 diabetes. Although it was not a complete surprise for Katja's mother, Natalia, since her father, uncles and grandmother all have type 1 diabetes as well, it was nevertheless unexpected.

"My husband and I decided to stop thinking about having another child. I was so upset that Katja had diabetes that I did not want to face the idea of having more children with diabetes," says Natalia, who hated the idea of her only child having to inject herself with insulin for the rest of her life. She remembers how her own father used to pack a special bag with all his diabetes paraphernalia whenever he had to travel.

"Now I know that I overreacted," admits Natalia, who is head of the accounting department at a nearby factory. "It is just a matter of paying attention. Katja and I have

no fears. We are now used to the lifestyle and we know how to take care of the diabetes." Natalia has several friends who also have diabetes, and she sees them living normal lives, marrying and having children. She believes there is nothing her daughter cannot do.

"I really don't think very much has changed since I was diagnosed with diabetes," says Katja. Her only objection is to the insulin injections and blood sugar tests, which sometimes hurt. In fact, Katja confesses that she does not check her blood sugar levels daily – she actually hates pricking her fingers and complains of swelling and discomfort. She checks her blood sugar only when she feels something is amiss and even that is rare.

"I know how to take care of myself. I've been doing it for six years now and it's easy," she continues. "I eat anything I want, but in small quantities. So I am the same as everyone else!"

Katja decided from the very beginning to look upon her diabetes as an adventure; something she must conquer. She regularly buys books to help her understand her diabetes and reads them diligently. She stays at the hospital for two weeks twice a year and makes the most out of her stays, meeting other children with diabetes, striking up friendships and listening attentively in diabetes school, where children are taught how to live with their diabetes.

"When I was first diagnosed, I took it very seriously. I was interested and wanted to learn. I was very responsible and made sure I understood everything. Now that I'm used to it, I sometimes get a little bit careless," she confesses, explaining that for a growing teenager diabetes takes second place in life.

Katja sees no point in being angry about her diabetes. After all, she cannot change the fact that she has diabetes and besides, she says, diabetes has brought a lot into her life. "Because of diabetes, I met Sasha and Tamara and other children at the diabetes hospital. Even though I have diabetes, there is nothing I cannot do. I have fun and go out with my friends. They all know I have diabetes, and it makes no difference to them."

Katja is well loved by her friends for her easygoing

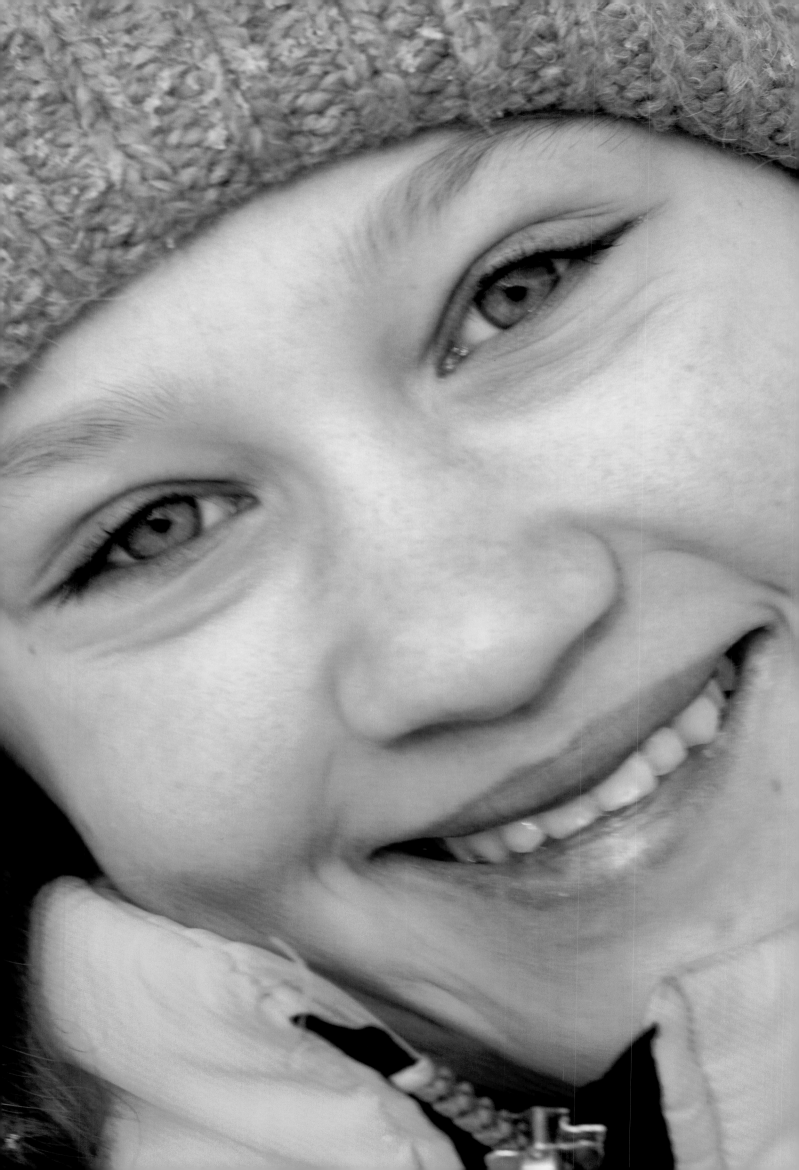

character, friendly nature and ready smile. The young girl has a penchant for collecting calendars featuring little children outlined in glitter by American photographer Lisa Jane. She tapes the calendars onto the mirror in her room and admires them several times throughout the day.

"I like pretty things! I like to draw and make jewellery and embroider, and these are all things that help me relax. When my sugar is too high or too low, I try to do things that make me happy so I can feel better," she says.

In school, Katja makes sure to attend gym class, even though she dislikes it.

"I like swimming and dancing, and I take walks every day so I can exercise, but gym is yucky," she exclaims, puckering up her nose at the thought of exercising at school. However, Katja knows the importance of exercising regularly and Natalia insists that her daughter has a healthy lifestyle that includes physical activity and good food choices.

"I truly believe that I am normal," insists Katja. "In Russia, sometimes people with diabetes are compared to drug addicts, because the addicts cannot live without their drugs and we cannot live without our insulin. But we are not addicts – we are normal. Addicts die from their drugs. But we survive and have better lives because of our insulin."

SASHA'S STORY

❚❚My blood sugar becomes high or low, and I feel sick and I regret being careless. I know my mother thinks I am not as good with diabetes as I was before, but sometimes I just forget!"

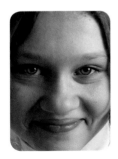

Sasha's blond curls, milky skin, rosy cheeks and sparkling eyes give her an angelic look. It doesn't hurt that she smiles constantly and loves to show affection. Her relationship with her mother is extremely close, so close in fact that Sasha relies on her mother, Irina, for all her diabetes needs.

"When Sasha was little, it was so much easier to regulate her blood sugar," says Irina, scolding Sasha, who is quick to blush. "Now, she is growing and I cannot watch her 24 hours a day, and she eats whatever she wants, sometimes without thinking. Then she comes to me and tells me she is not feeling well and I say, 'Huh! What did you eat today?'" Sasha squirms in her seat and avoids looking directly at her mother.

Sasha was always taught that nothing was forbidden, as long as her food choices were smart. Until recently she had a very active lifestyle including activities such as skating, swimming and snowboarding. Because she was exercising and burning calories, she could eat freely. Now hanging out with friends takes precedence over exercise, and the situation is very different.

"In many cases, parents suffer more than their children," says Irina. "They are more aware of how serious the disease is than children are. Sasha has lived with diabetes for so long that she finds it easy to cope with it now and does not think it's something to worry about, but she must never forget that it is in fact serious and must always be taken care of."

Irina cannot help but worry about her little girl. Sasha gave her parents quite a few scares when she was an infant. At the age of nine months she was mistakenly diagnosed with asthma and given antibiotics for almost ten months, switching from one course of antibiotics to another. Irina is convinced that the long period on antibiotics is what led to her daughter's diabetes.

"I work with doctors and I deal with infections and vaccinations, so I know something about the symptoms of diabetes," says Irina. When Sasha was four years old, Irina saw that Sasha had lost almost eight kilos in less than two weeks. She also drank a lot of water and made frequent trips to the bathroom. Irina thought of diabetes, but could not imagine that a child so young could have the disease.

"I think I was lucky to get diabetes when I was so young that I don't really remember it, because Mama says it was an awful time!" says Sasha, snuggling closer to her mother. "Mama says they took me to so many doctors and I was getting worse and worse, and no one knew what was wrong with me. No one even cared! Mama and

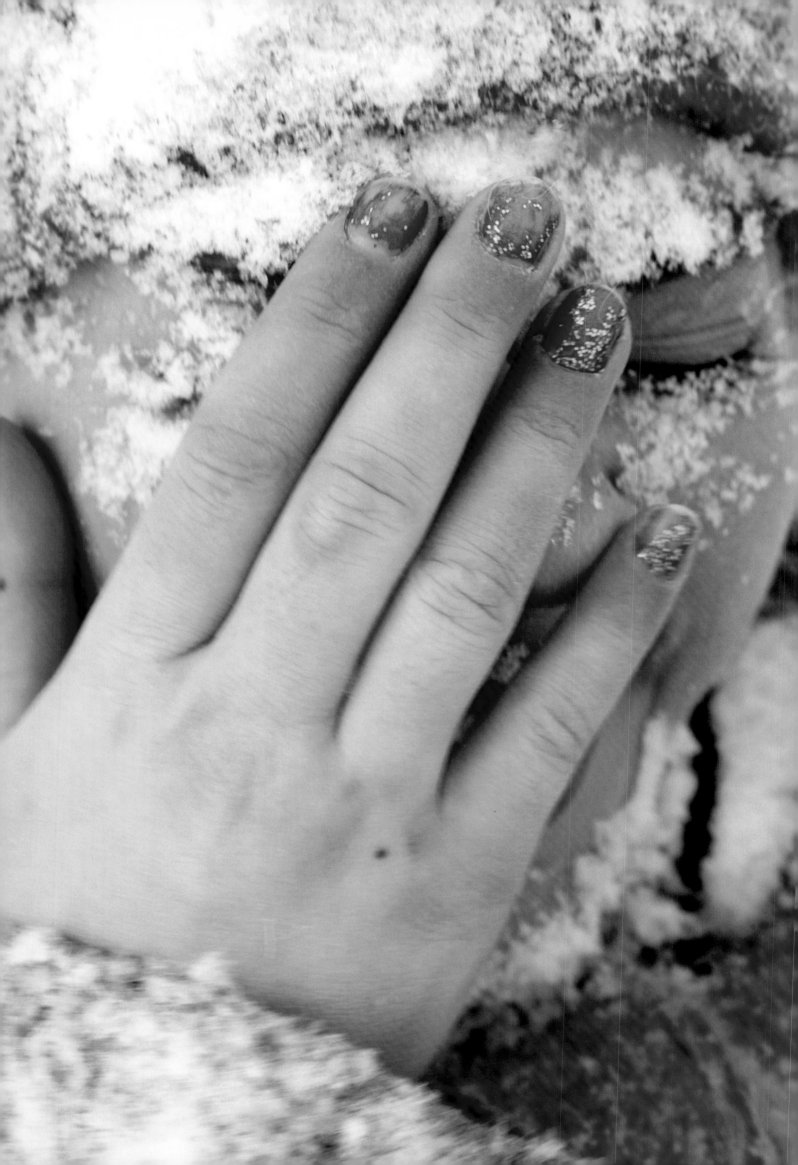

Papa took matters into their own hands and drove me to Yekaterinburg themselves, to the big hospital there, and demanded that a doctor see me."

Sasha was diagnosed with type 1 diabetes, leaving Irina devastated. Sasha, on the other hand, took it in stride, not minding the injections and returning to her naturally active and energetic self. However, it was difficult to find a kindergarten that would admit her.

"Things were tough in Russia at the time. People did not want to take on the responsibility of having a little girl with diabetes, which is considered a handicap in Russia," says Irina. "We could not find a kindergarten that would accept Sasha until she was almost six years old and able to take care of herself. By then, she was giving herself the insulin shots and I always gave her food to bring along. I didn't want her to have to rely on anyone else."

Today, Sasha's diabetes is a natural part of her life. Her days are dominated by school and friends. She loves to listen to music, play games on her computer and read her collection of fairytales, which she enjoys for their happy endings. She adores her cat, her stuffed animals and her 21-year-old brother, who is away at university in Yekaterinburg. She wants to be a vet. Diabetes has no place amidst all that.

"The only time I am reminded of diabetes is when I am careless and do not pay attention to what I am eating," says Sasha. "Then my blood sugar becomes high or low, and I feel sick and I regret being careless. I know my mother thinks I am not as good with diabetes as I was before, but sometimes I just forget!"

Like Katja, Sasha is admitted into hospital twice a year for a complete check-up, where she meets other children her own age who also have diabetes and learns even more about the disease. Surprisingly, Sasha's blood sugar levels are more regulated when she is at home with her mother than when she is at hospital on her own for two weeks.

"Well, in the hospital, I guess it's so much fun, like a big party with all us kids, and we go to the cafeteria and buy snacks and have feasts together. We hide it from the doctors and pretend we are low, so we need to have candy!" Sasha giggles at the memory, then smiles sheepishly at her frowning mother, who is shaking her head at her daughter. "I guess I am okay as long as my Mama takes care of me!"

TAMARA'S TALE

❚❚Mama got a book called *Diabetes – You and Your Child*. When I came back from hospital, and we were feeling depressed about what happened, we read a chapter every day and we began to see that we could cope with it. I saw that I had a lot of things in common with some of the stories in the book, and it wasn't so strange anymore."

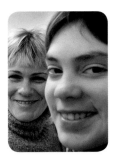

Tamara, a mischievous girl with a sense of humour, wants to be a hairdresser when she grows up, and her fashionable hairdo, long painted nails and colourful clothes are a testament to how much store she places in fashion. Although she sometimes appears older than her thirteen years, there are nevertheless moments of childishness, when Tamara laughs loudly as she romps in the snow with her dog. For Tamara, diabetes is even less of an issue than it is to the other girls.

A month before her diagnosis, then 10-year-old Tamara was stuck in an old elevator for forty minutes, and her mother, Lijuba, is convinced the horrible claustrophobic experience triggered her daughter's diabetes.

"Tamara started complaining of so many things – stomach pain, tiredness, hunger and then loss of appetite. She was always in a bad mood and never wanted to do anything. She was losing weight, too," says Lijuba. "One day, she went for a walk in the park with her father, and when they came back my husband said to me that something was wrong with Tamara because she drank two entire bottles of water in one go just out of the blue."

Tamara is a fiery mound of energy and her parents have often suspected her of being hyperactive. So when Lijuba came back from work one day and did not find Tamara

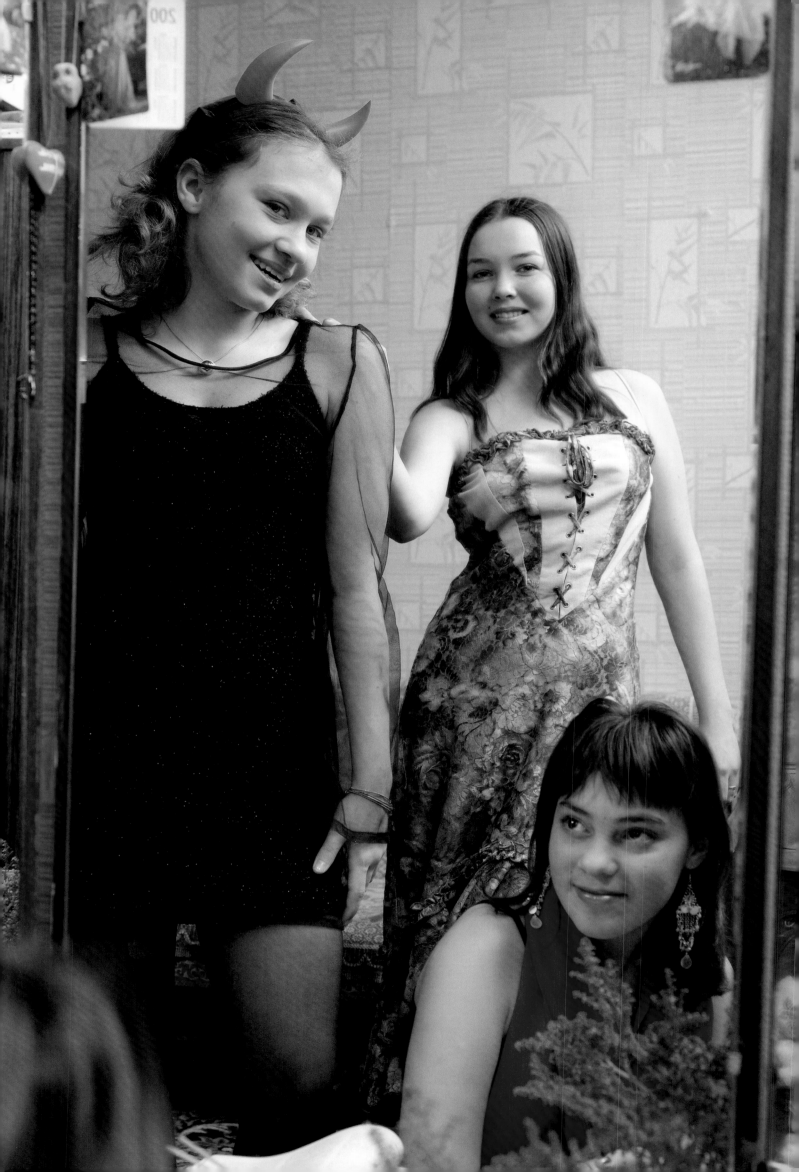

bouncing at the door to greet her, she was concerned.

"I found Tamara lying on the couch sleeping. I was so shocked! My daughter never sleeps during the day!" says Lijuba. "She was too weak to stand up so I called my friend, who is a paediatrician, to ask her for advice."

Lijuba rushed to the hospital with Tamara. When the doctors saw how weak the girl was, they decided to give her some glucose immediately, without bothering with any preliminary tests.

"She just got worse, and I was panicking," recalls Lijuba. "It was like she couldn't wake up. My friend arrived, and when she saw Tamara she made them stop the glucose and made them give her insulin instead. Within minutes, Tamara opened her eyes. I couldn't stop crying."

It was a stressful time for Tamara's parents, who were trying to appear as normal as possible in front of their little girl. Eventually, however, Tamara learned that she had type 1 diabetes.

"I was a little scared," says Tamara, admitting that she found it difficult to understand what was happening to her. "I cried sometimes, wondering why me, and what I had done to deserve it. But I stayed in hospital for two or three weeks where I learned a lot about diabetes."

Both Tamara and her mother began to understand more about the young girl's diagnosis, and the information began to make sense. They met other people with diabetes and spoke to them as much as they could so as to learn how to live with diabetes.

"Mama got a book called *Diabetes – You and Your Child*. When I came back from hospital, and we were feeling depressed about what happened, we read a chapter every day and we began to see that we could cope with it. I saw that I had a lot of things in common with some of the stories in the book, and it wasn't so strange anymore."

Slowly, Tamara began to accept the new addition to her life and refused to allow it to disrupt her rhythm. When she returned to school, she answered all her friends' questions about diabetes and Lijuba spoke to Tamara's teachers, informing them of her daughter's condition. Lijuba also spoke to all the parents of Tamara's classmates.

"It was a parent-teacher event and I announced to everyone that Tamara has diabetes. I told them that it is not an infectious disease and that their children would not catch it from my daughter. I asked them to explain to their children what diabetes is, so that no one would treat Tamara differently. I also wanted to tell the parents that they had to make sure their children were living a healthy life so as to avoid diabetes."

Tamara no longer wonders why diabetes had to happen to her. She believes that such things happen for no reason and there is no explanation for some things. She considers diabetes an excuse for her to lead a healthy life – one in which she plays basketball five times a week, counts her calories as much as possible and still has fun with all her friends.

"Diabetes does not restrict me in any way," says Tamara. "It just makes me more careful. It helps me. So the truth is; I should be grateful to it!"

MINOR FEARS AND TREPIDATIONS

IIThe thing is," explains Sasha, "No matter what happens to us, it is nice to know that we have each other to count on. It's true we never talk about our diabetes with each other – we don't get the chance to see each other that much and we don't want to waste time talking about diabetes! But if I ever need to talk to someone, I can go to Katja or Tamara, and it's the same for them. That's a nice feeling."

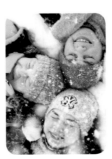

"They are optimistic, these girls. That's why they survive," says Irina, Sasha's mother.

"They are growing up and diabetes is becoming a little bit harder for them because their bodies are changing and their worlds are expanding, but they look

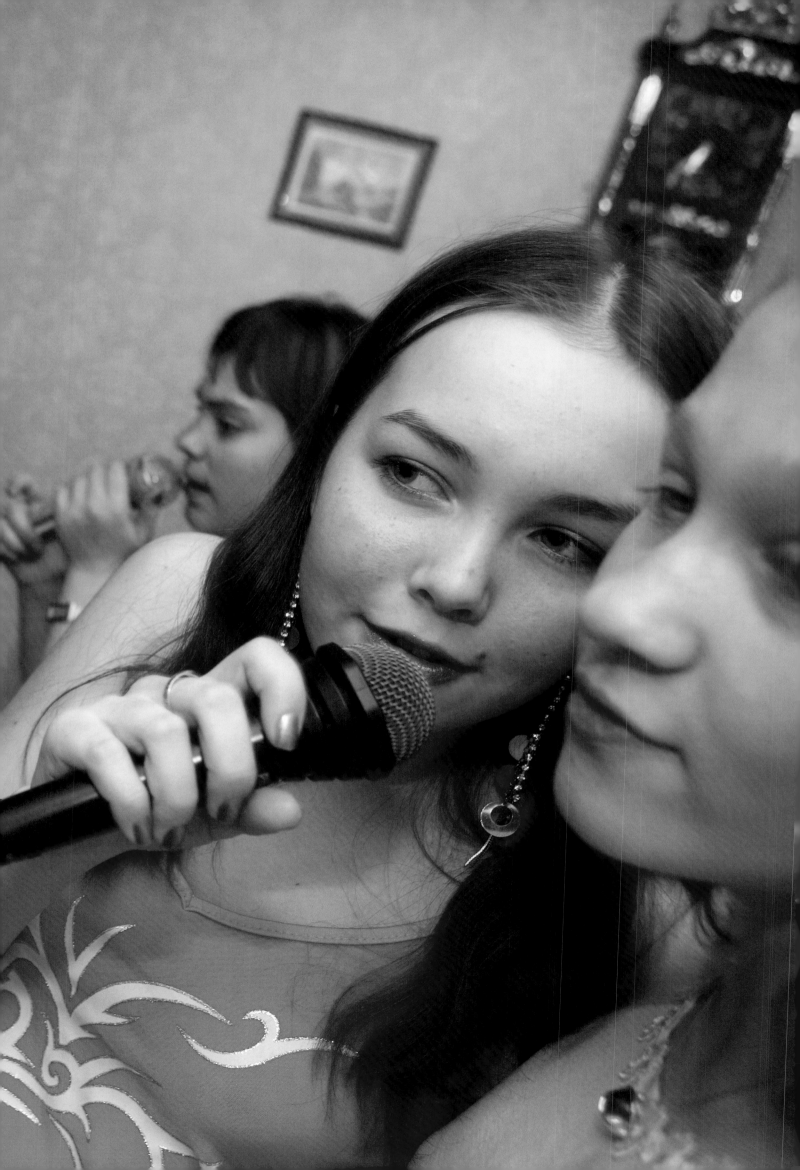

on the bright side and focus on having a good life. That is what helps them."

As Irina said, diabetes is becoming harder to handle for the girls as they grow up, and despite their cheerful nature, they do have a few personal worries.

Katja dreams of becoming a doctor, and knows she must go away to live at the university in Yekaterinburg to fulfil her dream.

"I have heard it will be very difficult there and that the schedule is intense. I will not have my mother there to support me. I am worried it might be hard and that I might find it difficult to regulate my blood sugar levels."

Sasha is afraid of losing the high level of diabetes care that she has now.

"In Russia, people under 18 with diabetes get the best the government has to offer. We get good insulin and regular check ups at the hospital and everything we need. After 18, we may no longer be given insulin cartridges for our pens and I may have to use syringes, which I have never used." Sasha and her friends are afraid they will no longer be regulated as well as they are now if their current therapy is stopped.

Tamara, on the other hand, has no idea what to expect of the future and is simply living in the moment. She is just entering her teens and the changes in her body are affecting her blood sugar levels.

"I am still learning what is best for me; what is the best way to regulate the glucose in my blood. But even so, I feel it is easier now than it was in the beginning, because I am getting used to it."

"The thing is that no matter what happens to us, it is nice to know that we have each other to count on. It's true we never talk about out diabetes with each other – we don't get the chance to see each other so often and we don't want to waste time talking about diabetes! But if I ever need to talk to someone, I can go to Katja or Tamara and it's the same for them. That's a nice feeling," says Sasha.

LIFE GOES ON...

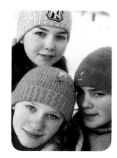 For now, the three friends and their mothers are thankful for how well they have all adjusted to life with diabetes. They have been able to achieve a good balance, and all of them have reached the conclusion that life is so much bigger than diabetes. Consequently, control is crucial and non-negotiable.

None of the girls see diabetes as something to be embarrassed about or ashamed of. On the contrary, all their school friends are very much aware of what diabetes is and what it entails.

"I told all my friends and explained to them that sometimes I might get very low blood sugar and have to eat a snack," says Sasha, waiting to hear what Katja will add.

"Yeah, me too. My friends always buy me something sweet if I need it, and Tolya is so sweet. He is always looking out for me and stopping me from eating too much chocolate!" Katja says, mentioning her boyfriend.

"My friends walk me home from school when I am not feeling well, so that I am never alone. They're so sweet!" says Tamara, playing with her tousled strands of hair.

Soon, the three girls become bored of the diabetes talk and begin a game of basketball instead. Tamara thrusts the ball at Katja, who grabs it with both hands and takes off running, hounded by a shrieking Sasha. After having chased each other for a while, the girls collapse on the floor.

They tire of the game quickly. They turn their attention to each other and with their arms intertwined the girls sit down on a bench, all three chattering simultaneously.

They have much to discuss: boys and music and clothes and movies and school. And boys. At this stage in their lives, diabetes is too insignificant for them to dwell on.

It is enough that it has brought them together.

Victor

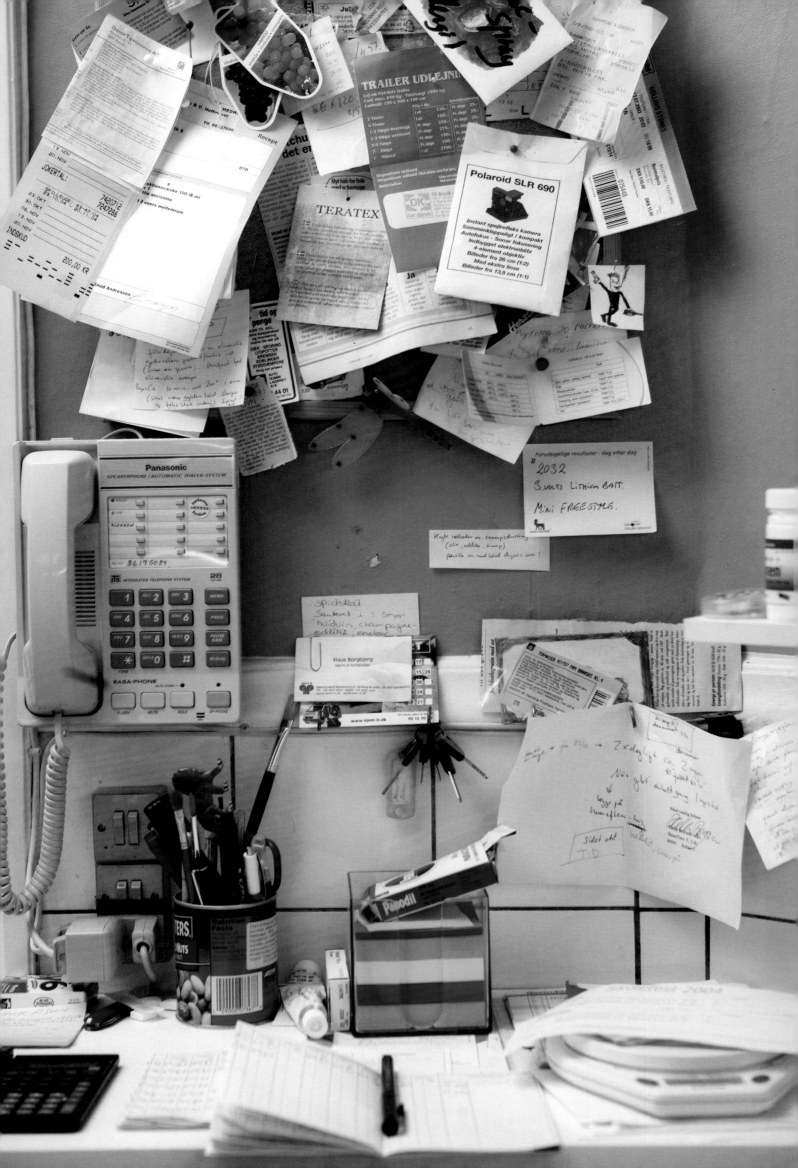

Victor Martin Jensen

Victor, a 10-year-old boy with type 1 diabetes, and his mother, Merete, are role models for every person who finds himself or herself in their situation. Every obstacle can be overcome by hard work, faith and fortitude, and the Victor-Merete pair is an excellent example of that sentiment.

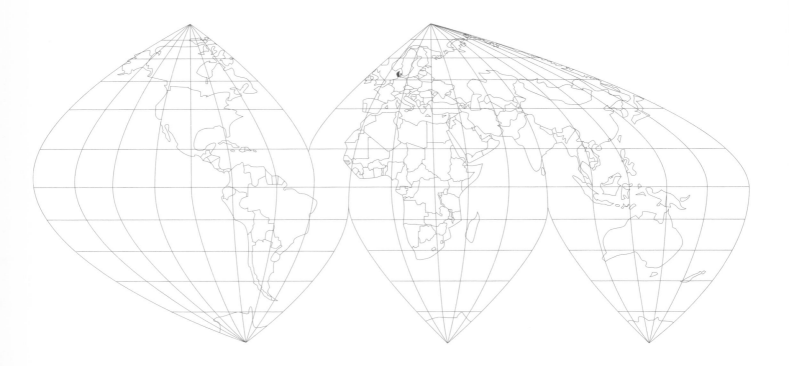

DENMARK

Situated in northern Europe, Denmark consists of the peninsula of Jutland – or Jylland – in the west, and an archipelago of more than 406 islands in the east. Denmark's highest point, which is Yding Skovhøj in Jylland, lies 173 metres above sea level.

The climate is cool and temperate, with rainfall throughout the year. Important sectors of Denmark's economy are agriculture, fishing and forestry. Some oil and natural gas is produced from fields in the North Sea. Denmark's main industries are iron and metal working, food processing and brewing, chemicals and engineering. Exports include machinery, food, chemicals, furniture, transport equipment and fuel and energy. [1]

STATUS Monarchy
POPULATION 5,432,335 [2]
PEOPLE WITH DIABETES 265,000 [3]
LANGUAGE Danish
RELIGIONS Protestant, Roman Catholic

[1] The country information is summarized from The Times Atlas of the World - Consice Edition, 1996.

[2] U.S. Census Bureau, International Data Base, September 30, 2004.

[3] International Diabetes Federation, 2004.

"I know now it is a situation, not a sickness."

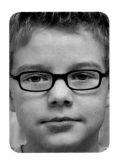

"I like this kind," he says as he finishes the last bit of his ice cream, oblivious to the chocolate dribbling onto his chin. Licking his sticky fingers clean, he eyes a plate of bakery-fresh pastries nearby.

"Mom, can I have one of those?" he asks, hypnotised by the pastries.

"Victor, it's either ice cream or the sweets, not both, you know that," sighs Merete, puzzled why her usually sensible son just cannot stop craving sugar this afternoon.

"I know that, mom! Wait!" He jumps out of his chair and runs to his bedroom to get his glucometer and test his blood sugar level.

A few seconds later he rushes back into the room, brandishing the glucometer high and thrusting it towards Merete to prove to her that it has confirmed what he already knows: his blood sugar level is still low, and he can afford to have some more sugar.

He grins and watches the pastry as it is moved from the centre of the table to the plate in front of him. Within a

few seconds, the pastry has disappeared, leaving behind a few clinging crumbs and a look of satisfaction on Victor's translucent face.

"You see, I don't have to say 'no' always. We'll just get punished later if we place too many restrictions on him," says Merete, smiling gently at her 10-year-old son.

DELAYED DIAGNOSIS

❚❚ He was losing weight. He was also going to the toilet a lot more, and he started wetting his bed. It just kept getting worse and worse and worse. It happened so often! I thought maybe we should take a sample of urine and go to the doctor."

'Gentle' is the word that instantly comes to mind when one thinks of Merete Breth Jensen. The young, working mother and her husband live in Århus, Denmark's second largest city, with their only son, Victor Martin Jensen. The family's small apartment is filled with photographs in antique frames, well-worn books with dog-eared corners, fresh flowers in simple vases and lazy cats napping in armchairs.

Their home's warmth, however, could not shelter them from the harshness of the unexpected. Two years ago,

Victor was diagnosed with type 1 diabetes and life as they knew it was turned upside down.

"It was a very warm summer. Victor was drinking a lot of water and he was always thirsty," Merete says, as she begins the story she has told so many times by now. "He was losing weight. He was also going to the toilet a lot more, and he started wetting his bed. It just kept getting worse and worse and worse. It happened so often! I thought maybe we should take a urine sample and go to the doctor."

Suddenly, her voice hardens, leaving no trace of her natural gentleness.

"We did that three times; three urine samples over a period of three weeks. And they couldn't tell us what was wrong. It took three weeks before we learned that he had diabetes. I was so angry. I still am! We could have spared him those weeks of pain."

After a blood test preceded by medical examinations that yielded nothing, Victor's parents were told he had type 1 diabetes – a disorder they knew nothing about at the time. Merete tried to understand what was going on, but was unable to comprehend the magnitude of the diagnosis.

The high level of glucose in Victor's blood was almost at the point of sending him into a hyperglycaemic coma. The medical team wanted to admit Victor to hospital immediately but, against the doctor's advice, Merete left the clinic to take Victor out for a meal at a popular fast-food restaurant. She did not realise that the sooner he had professional medical care, the better.

"We had to go, I couldn't let him down. I had promised him," she explains. "I don't think I understood the seriousness of his condition."

That day she picked up Victor's best friend, Johannes, and watched the boys play as they picked at their burgers and fries. She did notice, however, that Victor did not have as much energy as Johannes and his appetite was not as robust, but she felt she could not disappoint her son. After a nerve-racking afternoon, Merete and Victor returned home to pack a few things and headed to the hospital.

A CHILD'S EXPRESSIVE STROKES

❚❚ I like this present from Johannes. The alien is like me: different."

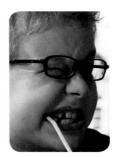

"I don't remember the hospital, but Mom was there," shrugs Victor, refusing to dwell for long on the five days he spent at Skejby Hospital, Denmark's second largest hospital, with his mother. "But I remember Johannes came to visit me and he brought me this," he says, scurrying off his bed, scattering stuffed animals onto the floor, to ruffle through a stack of loose papers and notebooks. A few seconds later, he pulls out a tattered comic book about a green alien. "I like this present from Johannes. The alien is like me: different," Victor tries to explain, proving his point by displaying several pages of illustrations featuring the green alien, all of them drawings he has made himself.

While other children might keep a diary, Victor draws to record his life; it is his own personal form of expression. "This is what I want to be," he says, pointing at a picture he once drew of himself wearing an artist's beret and stroking a canvas with a paintbrush.

He has titled the drawing 'Le Victor,' dreaming of the day his name will hold such artistic grandeur. Drawing, for Victor, is an escape. It allows him to relax and spend time alone in his room with his thoughts. Drawing is also his way of expressing the whirlwind of emotions he experiences daily while living with his diabetes. His feelings and trepidations are translated into the strokes of his brushes and the colours on the paper, erasing his frustrations, worries and fears.

Merete is proud of her son's budding talent.

"During the first year of his diabetes, most of his drawings were about food, candy and ice cream," says Merete, listing the types of food Victor was learning to reduce in his diet. He drew illustrations of a small child with glasses – strongly resembling himself – reaching

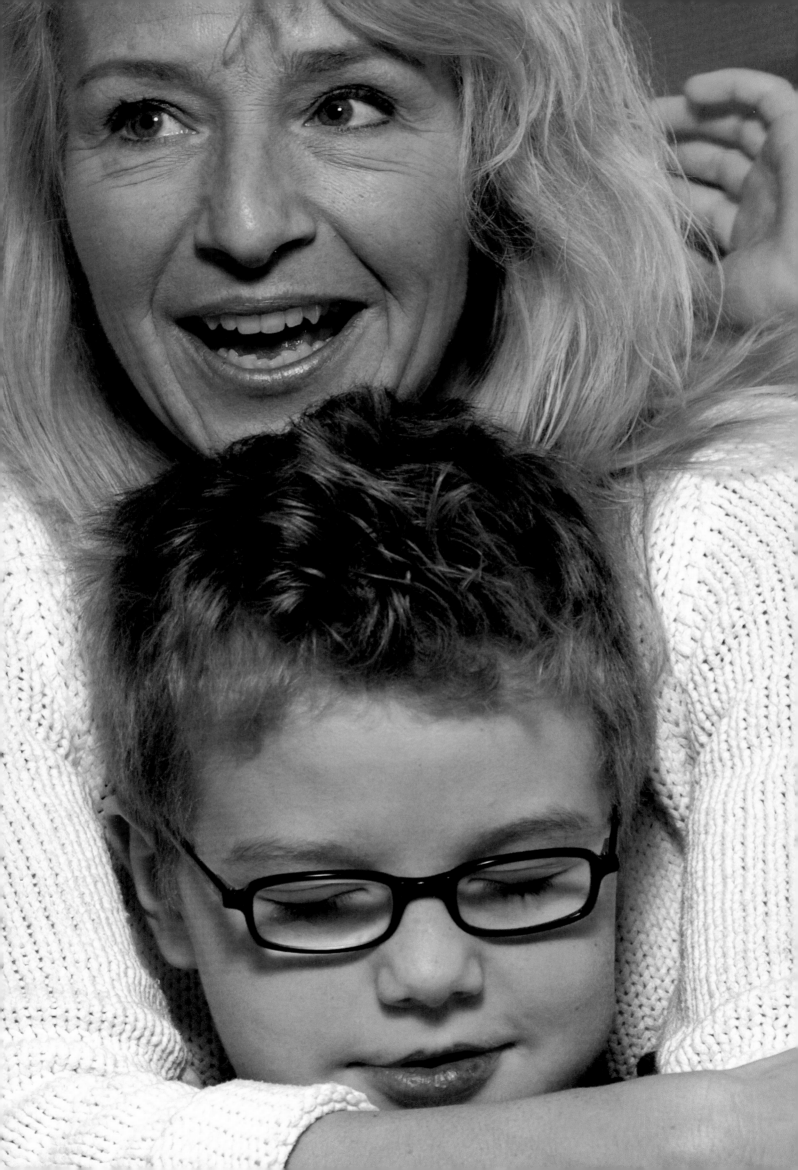

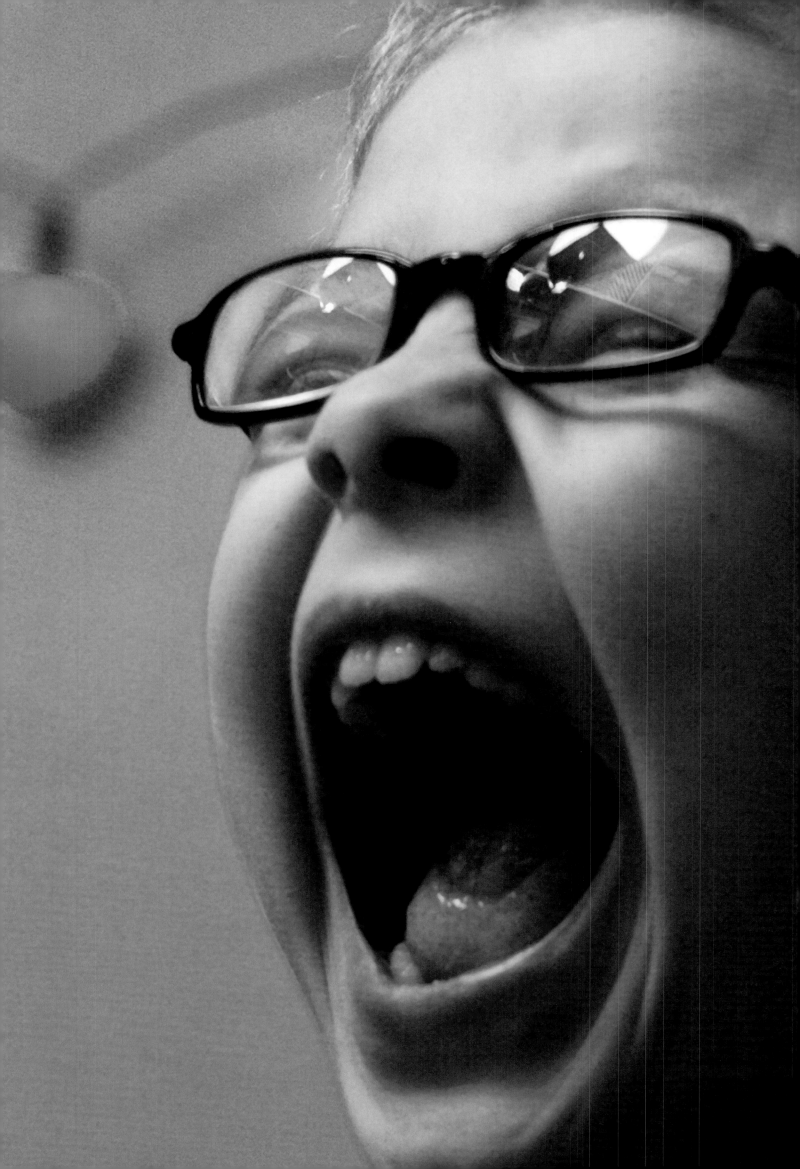

across a table towards a burger and fries meal and an ice cream sundae. In that drawing, the food is just out of reach of the little boy's fingers.

"Now I don't only draw food," Victor assures his mother. His drawings are varied in their subjects, ranging from quick sketches of his cat, Molly, to elaborately detailed murals of soldiers engaged in battle. Victor's imagination knows no bounds.

MERETE'S HIDDEN MISERY

❚❚ One day, I walked onto his school's playground and I thought to myself, 'There are 500 kids in this school, so why Victor? It's so unfair! I'm so angry!'"

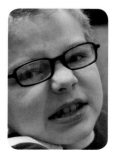

Victor's hospital stay does not hold horrible memories for him, but for Merete it was five of the longest and most confusing days of her life. It sometimes felt like the endless information she was given would never make sense to her. Everything was new territory, for Merete knew nothing about diabetes, despite the fact that two of her uncles had died of complications from type 1 diabetes.

The hospital staff made it very clear to Merete and her husband, Niels Jensen, that their son could not leave the hospital until they understood everything they needed to know about "this diabetes thing," as Merete calls it. Niels and Merete attended many workshops, talked to a range of specialists, learned about correct food choices from a nutritionist and listened to diabetes nurses. Finally, the family learned everything they needed to know.

In addition, Merete and Niels educated themselves by doing their own research – surfing the Internet and reading as many relevant articles as they could find. Victor, on the other hand, was too young to grasp what was going on.

"It was a misery; a very hard time for all of us," says Merete about the period during and several months after Victor's hospital stay. The confusion, anger and frustration she suddenly found to be a part of her life had begun

to affect her. She admits that she experienced bouts of depression at the time, when she finally buckled under the combination of exhaustion and panic. But regardless of what she was feeling, Merete never allowed Victor to see her tears.

"One day, I walked onto his school's playground and I thought to myself, 'There are 500 kids in this school, so why Victor? It's so unfair! I'm so angry!' Victor and I were angry together, but I never cried in front of him. I would cry to my colleagues at work, who were always there for me, but I had to be strong in front of Victor so that he could be strong himself."

WHEN WILL IT GO AWAY, MOTHER?

❚❚ I thought that when you got sick, you just went to hospital to get better and that was it."

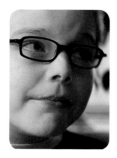

When Victor realised his insulin injections were not to stop, he began asking very personal questions. He found it hard to understand the disease – and that he would have it forever.

Today, he says that he never throws tantrums and never screams, complains or wails about his diabetes.

"But back then, I used to ask my mother, 'Why me? When will it go away?' I thought that when you got sick, you just went to hospital to get better and then you went home, and that was it." He pauses and swivels around on his desk chair, carefully choosing his next words. "That's why I always asked my mother, 'When will I be okay and when will the sickness go away? When can I stop taking the needle all the time?'" Suddenly, he is very still.

"Now I know it will never go away. It will always be there. Even when I am big."

Victor asked his mother that question – When will it go away? – a week after they returned from the hospital. It was a difficult question for her to answer.

"I would say to him, 'I cannot tell you, Victor. I do not know. Nobody knows. There's a lot of research being

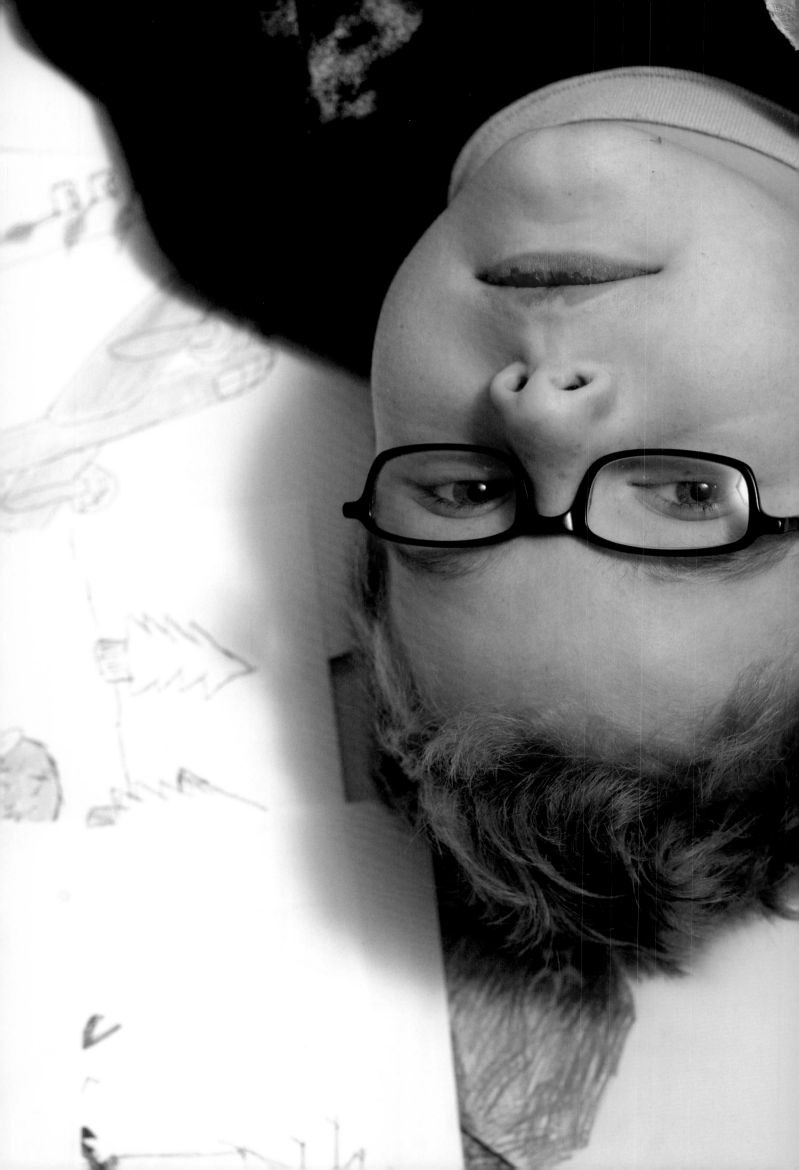

done and maybe one day they will be able to cure it.' I would also tell him that it was okay to be angry. He was very cooperative the whole time, and still is, but it's important for him to know that it's okay to be angry when he needs to be."

Merete has learned to come to terms with her son's diabetes. She is not angry anymore. She dealt with her anger by jotting down Victor's funny remarks or unique observations on scraps of paper she found lying around the apartment. Eventually, with the encouragement of her friend Elsebet, who advised her to try and be realistic rather than dramatic about Victor's diabetes, Merete's numerous scraps of paper were turned into a book.

The book is a very personal story told by a mother who has to tell her child that he is chronically ill. The story reveals what it is like to have a child with type 1 diabetes and advises other parents on how to deal with such a diagnosis. The book, which Merete calls her "contribution," is written in Danish. It is distributed throughout the country to all hospitals treating children with type 1 diabetes, so that their parents have a reference to fall back on. Although Merete had initially intended the book to be a comfort to other parents of children with diabetes, it also became a form of therapy for herself.

"Two years ago, when Victor was diagnosed, I desperately needed a book like this to guide me through, and I couldn't find one anywhere. Now I know I also needed to write it." The book, filled with Victor's detailed and expressive illustrations, is called *When will it go away, Mother?*

VICTOR'S VIEWPOINT

II Yes, it was unfair. Sometimes I feel angry, like when I am high or low. Sometimes the insulin injection hurts and other times I don't feel it at all."

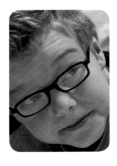

"Some days I don't feel I have it," says Victor, pausing from the Grand Theft Auto game he is playing on his computer. His tousled golden-blonde hair gleams in the fluorescence of his desk light, and he rubs his blue eyes beneath his thick glasses. "I know now it is a situation, not a sickness or disease. Some days I forget about it because I don't feel sick. But I can always tell when I am feeling sick, because when my blood sugar is high, I need to go to the bathroom and drink water. When it is low, I am tired and hungry and shaking."

He turns his attention back to his computer for a second, and then glances behind him to the small TV in his room, automatically tuned to the Cartoon Network. Apparently, a Tom and Jerry cartoon is about to start any minute now. "I tell my friends about it, the diabetes. Johannes knows a little, and Christopher at school also asks questions sometimes," he continues. "That's okay, I don't mind."

Slowly, he opens up further.

"Yes, it was unfair. Sometimes I feel angry, like when I am high or low. Sometimes the insulin injection hurts and other times I don't feel it at all."

Victor can administer the insulin injections himself; he finds it easy and is proud of his independence. He also tests his blood sugar himself, sometimes up to seven times a day, and is very much aware of what to do in case of a hypoglycaemic emergency, when his blood sugar levels are too low. He keeps a pack of sugar tablets made of pure glucose in the pocket of his pants at all times so that he can quickly and safely raise blood sugar levels that are too low.

Suddenly, he changes the topic.

"I like school, but I don't like the homework," he says holding back a giggle. "I like Danish class. English class too. I don't like math because it's hard sometimes. But I like the woodcarving class." With some coaxing, he admits that he also likes museums, aquariums, animals, sculptures and, most of all, swimming.

For Victor, swimming is a favoured hobby more than a prescribed activity. He finds comfort in the water, where he feels normal and in control.

"In the water, I feel free and light," he explains quietly. "Nothing else is important."

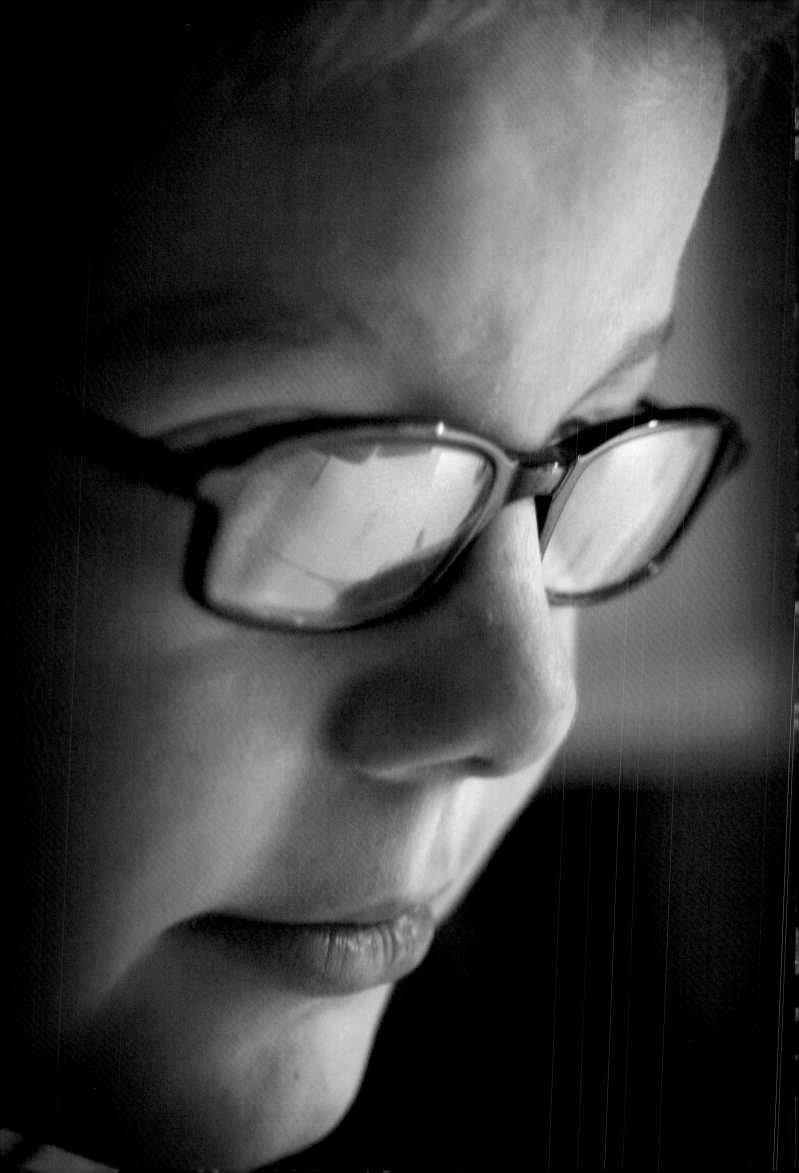

Victor is a sensitive, shy and imaginative youngster - an introvert like his father - who likes to spend hours alone in his room drawing pictures, reading comics and writing stories. Merete describes her son as a loner.

"Ever since he was quite small, he has enjoyed his own company. He doesn't need attention or to be around people all the time." She says it is not uncommon to find different types of 'Do Not Disturb' signs on his bedroom door. Merete has come across a number of them with warnings like 'Stay out, please!', 'I need to concentrate', or 'Girl Free Zone'.

In the early days after the diagnosis, she came across a sign that read, 'Keep Out, Especially You, Mom'. Merete smiles sadly when she recalls those early days.

"When he was first diagnosed, he took it out on me, of course, because I was the person closest to him."

Those days were short-lived, and Merete is now Victor's first refuge whenever he feels distressed, closely followed by Molly, his cat.

"Victor likes to just be with Molly. She is Victor's friend; she takes care of him and sleeps in his bed. I think she even sensed when he was sick because she always stayed so close to him."

Besides his faithful Molly, Victor cherishes a number of his possessions. First, there is Mads, the scrawny teddy bear he saw in a store window three years ago. Then there is the worn and tattered baby blanket usually wrapped like a scarf around his neck when he lies on his cushions watching his favourite cartoons. Victor also likes to spend time building with his Lego blocks. And finally, there are sheets of clean, crisp, white paper ready to be filled with the markings of pens, markers, pencils and paint brushes.

DIABETES SCHOOL:
NO LONGER ALONE ON A STRANGE PLANET

❚❚ Victor loves diabetes school and would love to have friends with diabetes. In fact, a boy has been diagnosed that Victor would like to get to know better – he thinks he can help him."

In the early months after Victor's diagnosis, the first – and only – edition of *I am Victor and I Have a Very Special Disease Called Diabetes* came out. It was a homemade newsletter, written and illustrated by 'Le Victor', and distributed to his mother and father.

"He wasn't happy with the diabetes at all, but he found his own way of dealing with it," Merete recalls. "While he sees himself as special, I don't think he wants others to see him like that. Still, he knows there are very few children who have type 1 diabetes, so he believes he *is* somehow special." Being 'special' is something Victor is very much aware of and expresses to his mother.

"Victor once said to me, 'Actually, I'm very rare, Mom, and Johannes says that I am too, because there are not many children who have type 1 diabetes like me,'" says Merete with a chuckle. "So you see, Johannes is confirming to him that he is special – a unique species!"

Though Victor understands that he is 'special,' he still feels lonely sometimes since he does not have any friends with diabetes. That's why he was thrilled to hear about the 'diabetes school' that he attends at a local hospital one day a week every other week.

This diabetes get-together currently brings together six children of roughly the same age who attend with their parents. The children talk about how they feel about having diabetes, share their experiences and learn from one other; the same goes for the adults.

Victor's excitement stems from his desire to meet other children "from the same planet," as he says. In fact, *Alone on a New Planet* is a subtitle Merete used in *When will it go away, Mother?*, and she admits that is how she felt two years ago when Victor was first diagnosed. However, she no longer feels so isolated.

"Victor loves diabetes school and would love to have friends with diabetes. In fact, a boy has been diagnosed that Victor would like to get to know better – he thinks he can help him. The boy and his mother are coming to visit us soon – the two boys are just about the same age, but this family have major problems because the boy will not accept the fact that he has diabetes. It's so awful for them. I really hope I can help them!"

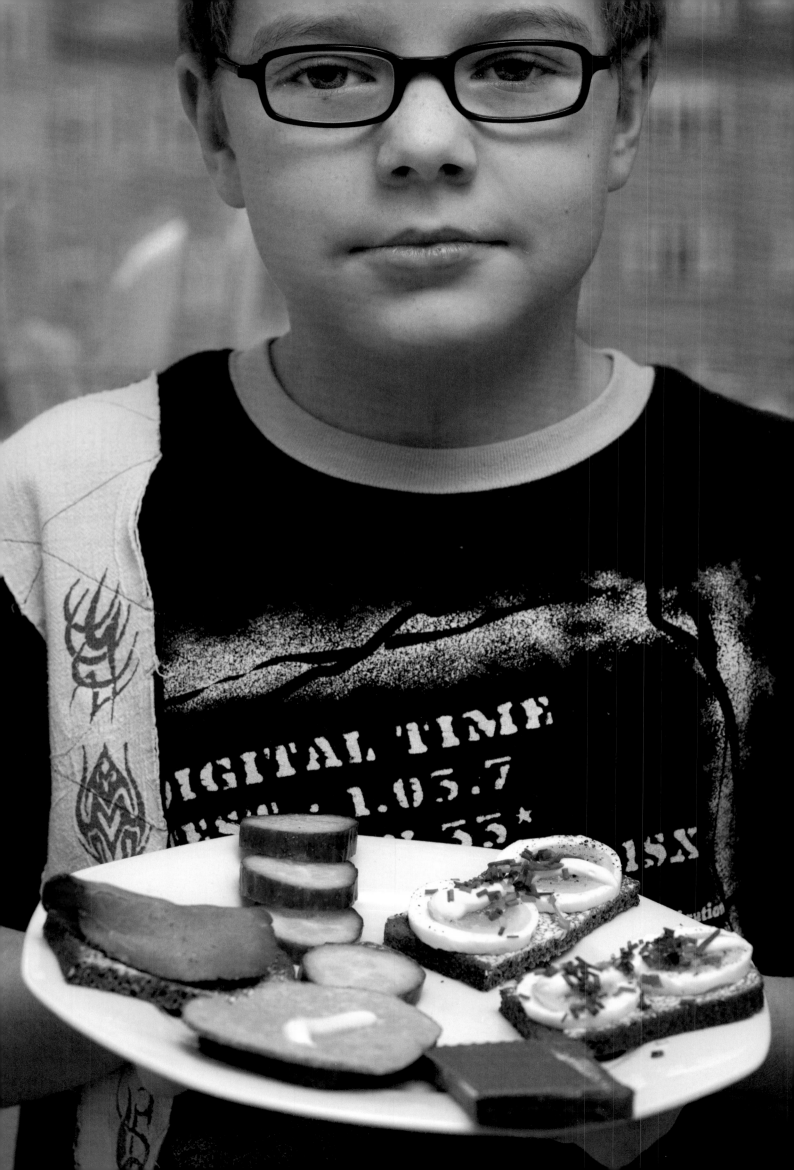

Merete is really passionate about helping other parents and young children diagnosed with diabetes.

"I want to write another book," she says. "I want to write one every two years, so we can help other families. Because we are one step further now, Victor, Niels and I, we are a bit more experienced and want to share our experience with others. It's becoming easier to understand and we're getting more relaxed about it too."

Diabetes, Merete realised, is easier to deal with when it is understood. Ensuring there is enough physical activity in one's life and taking greater care with what one puts into the body are the two major concerns as Merete sees it, and she has them covered.

VICTOR & MERETE;
RELYING ON ONE ANOTHER

❚❚Of course I'm worried about the future, even afraid sometimes. I will not always be there for him at the other end of the mobile telephone. In all this time, especially in the first year after the diagnosis but even now too, I have felt that the umbilical cord has been re-established between Victor and me. I want to hold him close all the time and protect him forever, but I cannot show him that."

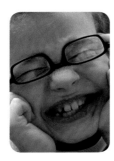

Victor is not as worried about his diabetes as his mother is and he does not yet completely understand why he has to check his blood sugar levels so often. Merete, however, wants to keep it like that for now.

"I'm not going to scare him. We don't talk about, you know, eye diseases and kidney diseases and problems with the feet and all those complications. His motivation right now is that he's feeling well. Because when he's high, he doesn't feel well, and when he's low, he doesn't feel well either."

She sees no reason to frighten the young boy; he is doing very well without anyone having to resort to threats. This perhaps explains Victor's reply when asked if he ever feels afraid.

"Afraid? Of what?"

"We are in control now. Diabetes does not control us," says Merete, her head held high and her eyes round with certainty. "I don't look upon his diabetes as a disease anymore, not really. Instead, I think diabetes is a good reason to have a healthy lifestyle.

"I heard a good phrase the other day," she says. "You don't die from diabetes; you die with it. It's a good one, don't you think?"

But despite her confident tone, Merete admits to moments of doubt. "Of course I'm worried about the future, even afraid sometimes. I will not always be there for him at the other end of the mobile telephone. In all this time, especially in the first year after the diagnosis but even now too, I have felt that the umbilical cord has been re-established between Victor and me. I want to hold him close all the time and protect him forever, but I cannot show him that.

"Instead, I do everything I can just to make him more self-confident. I tell him, 'You are just the best guy, Victor. You're so good! I am so proud of you!' I think it's very important to reassure your child." There is no doubt that Merete's patience and understanding have contributed immensely to making Victor the well-balanced child he is today.

Suddenly, a commotion is heard from her son's room down the hall. Victor bursts into the family room, giving a little skip and waving his glucometer underneath his mother's nose.

Merete gives the reading one quick glance and immediately jumps up.

"Oy, oy, he's low now," she explains, striding towards the freezer. Victor follows his mother eagerly, hopping from foot to foot, awaiting an unexpected treat. "Ah, Victor, this is because you didn't eat enough breakfast this morning," scolds Merete mildly. Victor grins and rips open the chocolate ice cream he is allowed to eat to raise his blood sugar level. The joy on his face says that there just might be some perks to 'this diabetes thing' after all.

Parojn

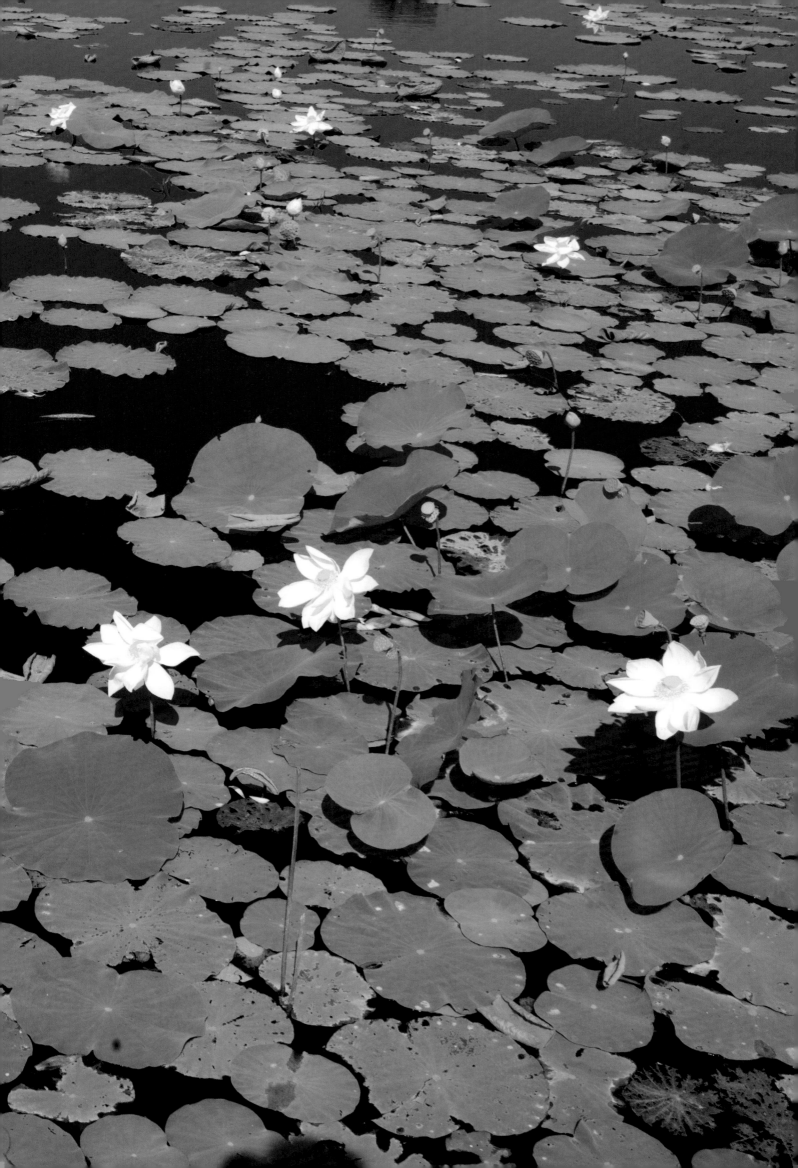

Parojn Chalermrojin

Each individual living with diabetes deals with this difficult situation in his or her own unique way. Young Parojn, living in the whirlwind that is Bangkok, exemplifies that. Parojn is learning how to live with diabetes at his own pace, with the gentle guidance of his parents. Day by day, he is gaining the confidence and know-how to fight back. In his own way, Parojn will soon be ready to grip the reins of his diabetes and steer his own course, with self-assurance and gratification.

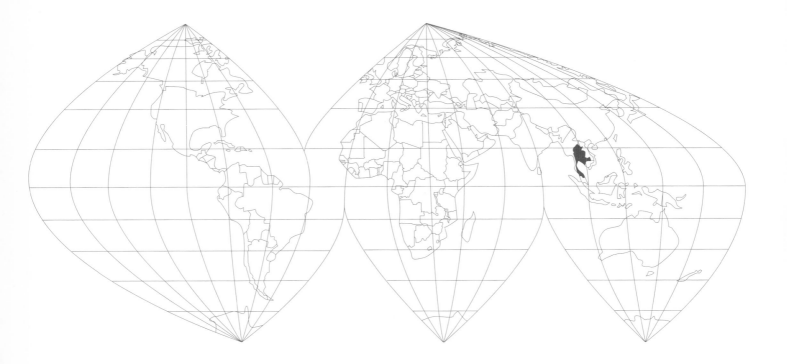

THAILAND

Thailand is bordered on the west and northwest by Myanmar, on the northeast and east by Laos and Cambodia, and on the south by the Gulf of Thailand, peninsular Malaysia and the Andaman Sea. The country's main river, the Chao Phraya, dominates central Thailand and the capital of Bangkok, the country's largest city and financial centre. The climate is hot and humid.

Agriculture occupies half of the workforce, and the main exports are rubber, rice, maize and tapioca. Fish and fish processing are also important. Thailand produces natural gas, oil, lignite, tin, tungsten and gemstones. Manufacturing of electronics, textiles, clothing and footwear is the most important contributor to the national income, while tourism is crucial as a source for foreign exchange.[1]

STATUS Monarchy

POPULATION 65,444,371 [2]

PEOPLE WITH DIABETES 1,536,000 [3]

LANGUAGES Thai, Lao, Chinese, Malay, Mon Khmer

RELIGIONS Buddhist, Sunni Muslim

[1] The country information is summarized from The Times Atlas of the World - Consice Edition, 1996.

[2] U.S. Census Bureau, International Data Base, September 30, 2004.

[3] World Health Organisation Web site, 2000 www.who.int

"Why can't I, why? Why only me?"

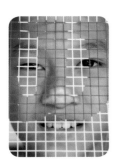

First, she wipes his skin clean with a little piece of cotton soaked in alcohol. Then she pinches the skin lightly, grasping a bit of flesh between her thumb and forefinger. In her other hand, the insulin pen is ready, prepared with the correct dosage. Slowly, she inserts the tiny needle at the head of the pen into the flesh of his arm, administering his second insulin shot of the day.

He does not flinch, his concentration focused on the bowls of food before him. Steamed brown rice, stir-fried tofu with green Thai vegetables, a fried egg with herbs and a small portion of wild mushroom soup are his dinner for the day, and he wants to get started as soon as possible. Hunger for a 10-year-old boy cannot be long lasting.

Parojn eats his dinner slowly and quietly, while his mother, Ratee, puts the insulin gear back into the small red bag. The young boy watches his mother out of the corner of his eye, but remains more interested in his food than in anything else.

Dealing with the insulin gear is Ratee's responsibility, not Parojn's. Although Parojn was diagnosed with type 1 diabetes about five years ago and has been living with

it for half of his life by now, he still refuses to administer the vital insulin himself.

"I am not afraid of the diabetes or of the injections," he says, shrugging his shoulders. "Sometimes they hurt and sometimes they don't. I'm used to them now. But I don't want to do it yet – stick the needle in me, I mean. My mother does it for me and she is teaching me, but right now I like it better if she continues doing it. I test the blood sugar levels myself, and I do it twice a day. That's my responsibility. But not the injections. I don't do them."

THEIR PRIDE AND JOY

❙❙He has to accept it and live with it – there is no other way."

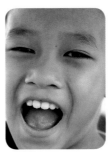

Parojn Chalermrojin is Ratee's and Preecha's only child. The couple looked forward to having this long-awaited child that they thought would complete their lives. When Ratee finally learned she was pregnant, the couple's excitement was only heightened by their preparations to welcome the new addition into their home.

But when he was five, their cherished Parojn suddenly began to look ill. He was losing weight quickly and his trips to the bathroom became abnormally frequent.

Eventually, he began to vomit regularly and, consequently, refused to eat. Because he continued to lose weight, he went into a spiral of severe exhaustion. His doting parents were instantly alarmed.

Parojn was rushed off to a hospital on the outskirts of Bangkok, Thailand's capital, where the Chalermrojins lived. He was quickly diagnosed with type 1 diabetes by the local doctor. His parents were not taking any chances. They took their boy to a private hospital that was quite a distance from their home, but where diabetes specialists could care for their son.

Parojn was admitted into the hospital for two weeks. For Preecha and Ratee, the shock was crippling. They could not bear the injustice that their only child was sick with an illness that would last for his entire lifetime. As Preecha admits, the knowledge of it was almost impossible to accept.

"The fact that it took us so long to finally have this son that we had longed for so much made it seem all the more unfair. Why Parojn, out of all children?"

Parojn's parents knew nothing about diabetes before their son's diagnosis, despite that fact that Ratee's mother as well as other relatives on her side of the family have type 2 diabetes.

They soon learned more about diabetes and how to take care of their son through the information given to them by the doctors and nurses at the hospital. The hospital also gave them a book about diabetes that provides suggestions for activities for Parojn, as well as tables and charts that can be used to monitor his blood sugar levels. Preecha and Ratee also use this book to explain Parojn's diabetes to his teachers at school, to ensure that the teachers are aware of and informed about their son's condition. Preecha also turned to the Internet and library books to learn as much as possible about his son's diagnosis. But regardless of all the information they were given and found themselves, the Chalermrojins were overwhelmed by the situation.

"At first, it was so hard to believe," says Preecha, sitting ramrod straight in his chair, his hands clasped in his lap and his wife sitting silently by his side. "Today, it is much easier to accept for the simple reason that we have to acknowledge it. This is what we have to tell our son constantly. He has to accept it and live with it – there is no other way."

At first, Parojn had a difficult time understanding his diabetes. The question 'why' never left him for long; he consistently asked his parents why he was stuck in a hospital, why he was being injected throughout the day, and why he could not have ice cream whenever he wanted.

"What can we tell him but the truth?" asks Preecha. "We truly don't know. And that's what we have been telling him ever since."

NOT READY TO DO IT ALONE

❚❚I am teaching Parojn to accept it."

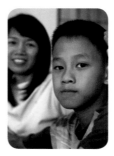

The heap of rice on his spoon is getting smaller and smaller and Parojn's attention drifts away from his meal. His ears prick up at the sound of shrieks and squeals outside; his friends from the houses next door are calling to him, urging him to join their games. He fidgets in his seat, clamouring to run out the door. Ratee, however, will have none of that.

"Finish your meal! You didn't eat enough," she says, admonishing her squirming son. "If you don't eat enough, your blood glucose will become low, so eat until I say it's enough!" Parojn obeys his mother without question – in fact, obedience is a characteristic both his parents are thankful their son possesses. The young boy ploughs through his meal, one eye on his mother, the other locked on the door. His mother knows best and Parojn knows it, so he will do as she says.

"Even when she cooks food I don't like to eat, I know I have to eat it because it is healthy and she has worked hard to prepare it for me," says Parojn. "And when I just want to go play, I know I have to listen to my mother and have a snack first, because we are always taking care of the blood sugar level, and I have to eat since I will burn

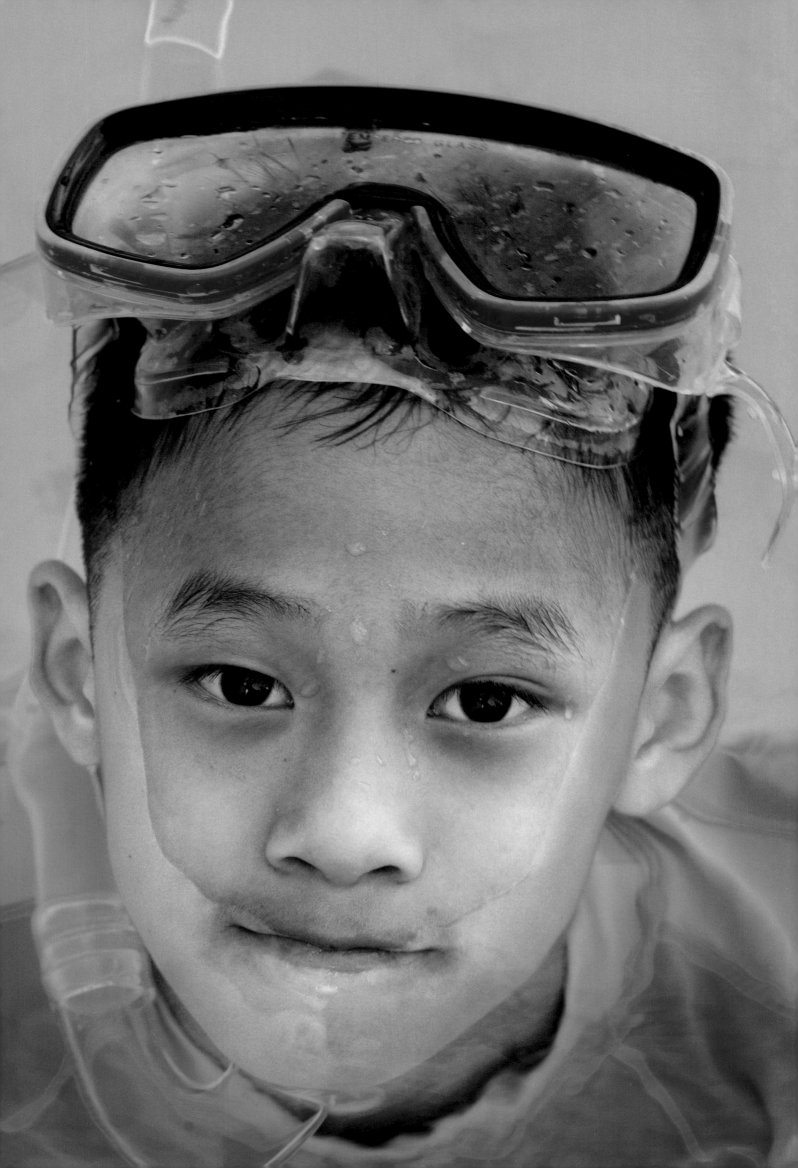

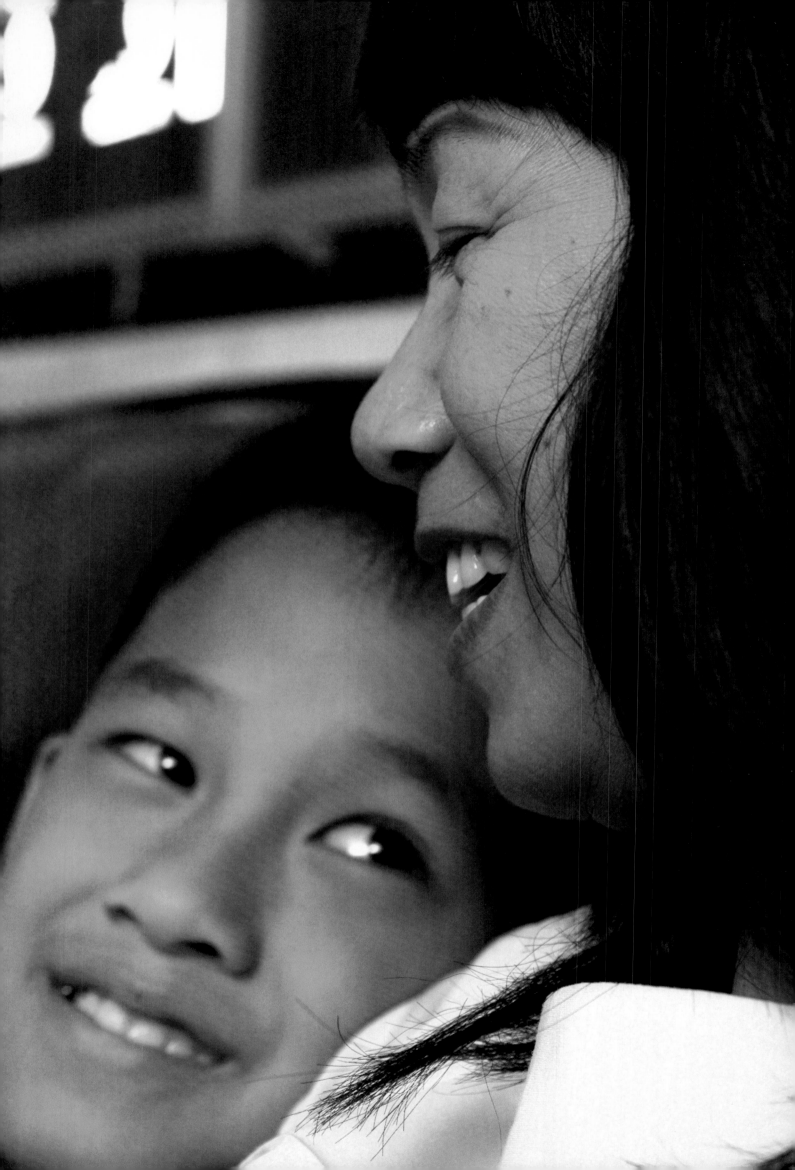

sugar when I play. I just wish there didn't always have to be so much planning."

Although Parojn does ask questions about his diabetes and takes some interest in it, it is clearly more of an issue for his parents to deal with – especially his mother. The young boy relies solely on his mother to manage his diabetes. She alone administers his daily shots of insulin. Preecha presides over these occasions, but prefers to leave the needle pricking to his wife.

"JingJo is very attached to his mother, yes," admits Preecha. Nong JingJo, or JingJo for short, is Parojn's nickname – a name he is more familiar with than the formal 'Parojn.' "Our son means the world to us, so we cannot help but be very protective of him. And for JingJo, his mother is essential for the management of his diabetes. Without her, he cannot take care of himself that well. He needs her for the insulin."

The close ties between Parojn and his mother are obvious. When she calls to him, patting the space on the couch next to her, he joins her instantly. He snuggles close to Ratee and her arms surround him. Her one hand alternates between rubbing his back and ruffling his hair, while her other hand entwines itself amongst his fingers. The two rest their heads against one another, with Preecha only a few inches away. Warmly engulfed, Parojn watches his favourite cartoon.

"I panicked so much when I realised that my son had diabetes," says Ratee, "And it will stay for his entire life! I kept asking myself, 'What will this mean for him?' But I accept it as a reality now, and I am teaching Parojn to accept it too. We have a special connection between us. Just a few words are enough for us to know what the other is feeling and that tie helps me so much in helping him."

That special connection manifests itself in many other ways. Two rooms make up the second floor of Parojn's home. One room is dominated by a queen-sized bed and a thick mattress on the floor. The other is quite bare except for an old refrigerator, a single-sized bed frame and stacks of storage boxes. The bare area is Parojn's discarded room, since he prefers to sleep with his mother.

Parojn's father chuckles as he describes the situation, briefly shaking his head. "He still sleeps with us, on the bed with his mother, while I sleep on the mattress! We tell him: 'Let's decorate your room and prepare it for you and you will have your very own room.' But JingJo says, 'No, thank you! There are ghosts in there and I prefer to stay with you.' He just doesn't like to be alone."

Parojn does not mind the lack of privacy, for the entire house is his playground. He does his homework at a desk in the living room. The couch provides a perfect place for reading comic books, watching cartoons and playing video games. The computer on its special desk, also in the living room, is handy for even more games, while right next to it is the musical keyboard where Parojn practices his piano lessons. Drawing can be accomplished on any old surface, and the rest of the time is dedicated to burning off his excess energy, whether on his old but sturdy scooter or while playing table tennis with his father or kicking a soccer ball around with his friends. Parojn says: "What do I need my own room for?"

PAROJN'S POSITION

"I know I am different."

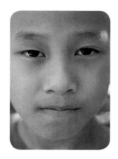

"I don't like this diabetes. I wish it would go away, but I know it won't. And I don't like it because it makes me feel different from all my friends," says Parojn, showing a little bit of the frustration his parents say he experiences every once in a while. "When I feel that I am so different, my father shows me pictures of other children with diabetes from all over the world. He tells me their stories, which he got from the Internet and I guess that makes me feel better. I am not alone, I know that, but sometimes it feels as if I am."

As Parojn grows up and approaches his teens, his shyness about his diabetes seems to be increasing. As a young child, he accepted diabetes as a normal part of his life. Talking about it posed no problems and Parojn never minded when his friends gathered around to watch Ratee inject him with insulin. After learning a bit about diabetes and what it meant to have it, Parojn's friends would quickly lose interest and return to their games.

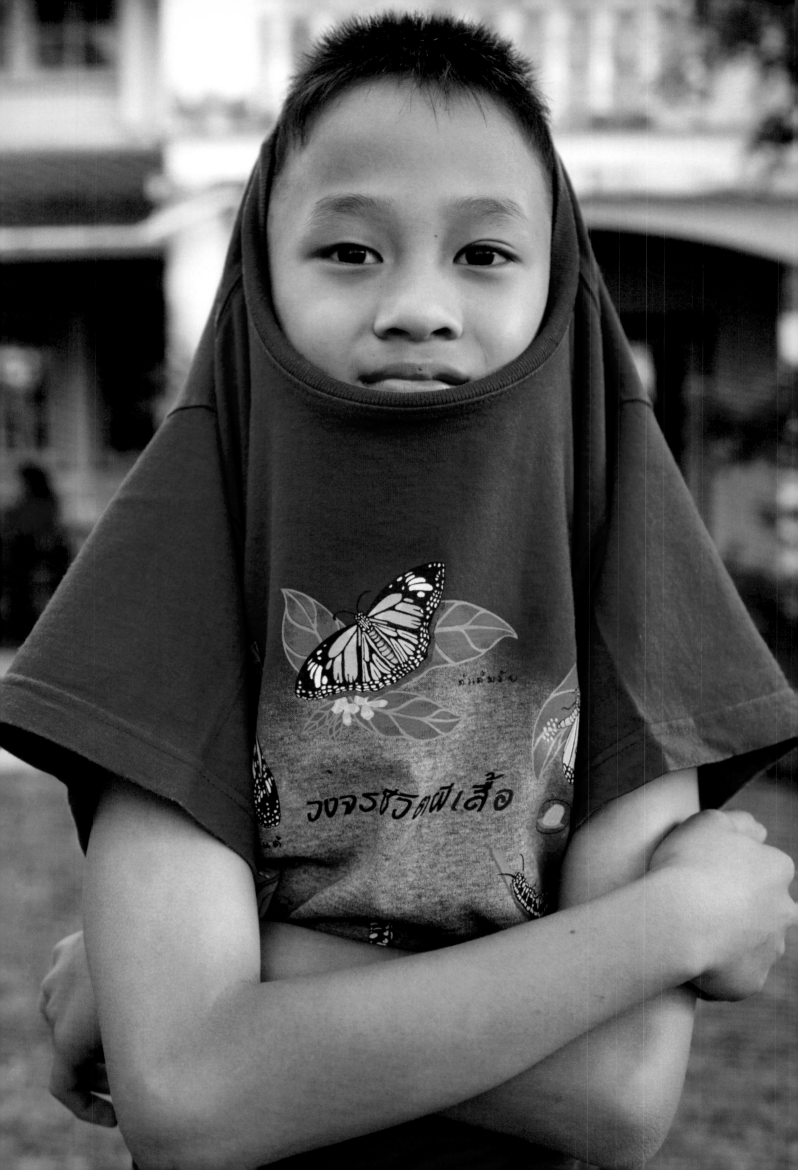

Recently, however, Parojn has started to hesitate in the car when the family heads out to a restaurant. He would prefer it if his mother would give him his insulin shot in the privacy of the car, away from curious eyes, before going into the restaurant. As he matures, diabetes is becoming a burden that he thinks makes him different from his peers. And Parojn resents that difference.

"I know I am different because I can't eat the same things as my friends," he says, pulling up his loose pants on his slight frame for the umpteenth time. "I always see the other children eat anything they want, but I have to ask my mother first and we have to figure out if it is alright for me to eat something at a specific time during the day, and we have to measure the blood glucose and think about it, and most of the time I can't eat things like candies and sweets. So I think to myself, 'Why can't I, why? Why only me?'"

Preecha and Ratee try not to restrict Parojn more than they have to, hoping to instil in their son a sense of acceptance. But as he grows, he resents the constant need to control what he eats. Food is always a priority and having to finish his food before going back to play is a nuisance that he particularly associates with diabetes. Though Parojn can't help but emit a tiny 'why?' underlined by an almost whispery whine every now and then, his mother says he does it more out of habit than anything else.

Parojn's parents work hard at remaining one step ahead of him, providing him with regular snacks throughout the day. "We try to be ready for him, so when he is hungry, there is something healthy at hand for him," explains Ratee. Furthermore, those little snacks are necessary to regulate his blood sugar levels, which are always fluctuating because of Parojn's high energy level.

In fact, to describe Parojn as having a lot of energy is an understatement. The 10-year-old barely sits still, rocketing through the house with his friends at his heels. After playing badminton for hours outside in the humid heat, he bounces back inside to wash his hands and grab a few slices of the guava fruit his mother had laid out for him. This particular fruit, she explains, is very high in vitamin C, and Parojn eats it with delight, all the while bouncing up and down on the couch.

DIFFICULTIES WITH DIABETES

❚❚For us, diabetes is a constant learning process."

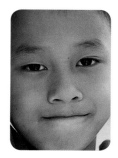

"We feel Nong JingJo is doing very well with his diabetes and we are very proud of him," says Preecha, thankful that his son listens seriously to his parents' advice. "He accepts what he is told and rarely makes a fuss about anything. Even if his mother makes him some food he doesn't like, he will eat it when she explains to him that it is healthy and will be good for him and his diabetes. His good-natured character makes it so much easier."

Nevertheless, Preecha and Ratee admit that some aspects are just out of their control, specifically their tireless attempts to control Parojn's blood sugar levels.

"JingJo's doctor is experimenting with a new approach regarding my son, so we are switching to a new type of insulin that we have to administer three times a day instead of the two times a day we were used to," says Preecha. Ratee gives Parojn his first insulin shot of the day when he wakes up, then again in the afternoon before the evening meal, and finally at night just before he goes to bed. Because of this new regimen, there are major fluctuations between Parojn's 'highs and lows'. He is always either too high, meaning his blood sugar levels are more than they should be, or too low, meaning his blood sugar levels need to be brought up either with some glucose tablets or with sweet fruits.

"For us, diabetes is a constant learning process," says Preecha. "Ratee sometimes worries a lot when she sees that Parojn's sugar level is too high and there is no explanation whatsoever. But we know that all we can do is to try and regulate it and increase our understanding of the disease. We are still learning, even after five years."

Parojn's parents are constantly reminding him that his diabetes will remain with him forever and that he therefore has to learn how to take care of himself properly. They will send him to diabetes camp in six months, where he will spend five days with other children with diabetes, learning about diabetes from professional nurses and doctors and, most importantly, hopefully find the courage to inject himself. "We are not putting pressure on him right now. Let him test his own blood sugar and let his mother give him the shots. When he is ready, he will do it himself," says Preecha.

Though hyperactive and in constant motion, Parojn can also be a quiet boy of few words. He chooses the words to describe his feelings very carefully. "When I go to diabetes camp and meet other kids who have not had diabetes as long as I have, I will tell them not to worry. If they can find something that brings them comfort, it will be so much easier for them and not hard at all. For me, the insulin injections are a bit hard and control of the blood sugar levels is hard too, but I keep trying with my mother and father and it is actually becoming easier. I will share that with the other kids to make them feel better.

"I want to have more friends who have diabetes so I won't feel all that different," adds Parojn, admitting he is looking forward to going to diabetes camp. "I don't think I will be afraid anymore of giving myself the injections. I know I have to learn to do it over there." His worry at the moment is that he has to be away from his parents, especially his mother, for five days. He has never spent a night away from her in his life and going off to camp is a big step for the young boy.

ACTIVITIES AND INTERESTS; LIFE BEYOND DIABETES

▐▐As long as I am careful, I can do all the things I like."

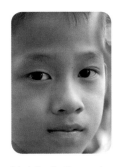

Day by day, Parojn is learning that diabetes does not mean his freedom has been taken away from him. He can rush off to play at his friends' homes as long as he has a snack to compensate for all the sugar he will burn. He can ride his bike in the park, spend a day window-shopping with his parents at the mall before going to the food court or run on the treadmill if he feels like it. He can engage in all the activities and interests he enjoys, as long as he is cautious and aware of his needs.

"I like swimming, snorkelling, bird-watching, camping and playing tennis, and I can do all these things as much as I want! I don't feel sick, but I know that I may become sick if I am not careful. As long as I am careful, I can do all the things I like, so I do not have to feel sad about having diabetes," says Parojn.

Parojn and his parents often take off to Tung Salaeng Luang National Park on weekends to camp and spend time together in the beautiful countryside of northern Thailand. Parojn cherishes these weekends, where he can do whatever he wants. The family take long hikes in the forests, swim and fish in the streams, take pictures of strange flowers and insects and spend hours bird watching, their favourite pastime.

For the past three years, bird-watching has been a serious hobby for Parojn and his father. They share a professional telescope and a strong pair of binoculars and enjoy spotting some of Thailand's more than 900 different bird species. "We have this book: *The Birds of Thailand*," says Parojn. Many of the birds in the book are highlighted or circled, signifying that they have been spotted by father and son.

"And look, this bird is called the Yellow-vented Bulbul and it always comes to our garden around May and June, because there are lots of insects at that time! This bird built a nest in our tree last year, and it was so much fun watching it!" Every time the young boy spots a new bird, he runs to fetch his book and look it up, eager to learn all about it.

Diabetes has never hindered the family from embarking on these trips. They simply ensure that they bring along extra vials of insulin to use if needed, and they try to take things nice and easy. Parojn is truly free during these trips, when his diabetes takes a step back so he can give his sensitive nature free reign. He whispers gently to his favourite plants and animals and paints beautiful watercolours of the birds he loves to observe. For Parojn and his family, this is a healing environment.

Parojn describes activities like bird-watching and swimming as "beautiful; things of comfort." Those calming activities soothe him. "The feeling I get when I am doing these things that I love is the same feeling I get when I am upset about diabetes and I go to my mother. She gives me comfort and I feel better, just like when I am watching the beautiful birds and swimming in the water."

A MOTHER'S WISDOM

❚❚'Things could be much worse.' We are thankful at least that he has something that can be controlled as long as we pay attention and are careful."

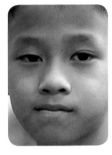

Ratee's life revolves around her son. She sends him off to school in the morning and waits for him to return in the afternoon, ready to take care of him until he goes to bed at night.

"I was very shocked when I first learned about his diabetes and it was so, so hard to accept. Maybe that is why I remain overprotective. But things are getting easier and easier each day, and I am worrying less and less. Still, the worrying will never go away completely."

When Ratee takes Parojn to the hospital for his check-ups every two months or so, her heart aches at the sight of babies not more than three or four months old who have been diagnosed with type 1 diabetes. She cannot help but feel lucky that her own son was diagnosed when he was five years old, at a time when he was able to understand the condition and work with his parents to control it.

"I see all the sick children in the hospital, suffering from awful diseases and I think 'Things could be much worse.' We are thankful at least that he has something that can be controlled as long as we pay attention and are careful."

Ratee acknowledges that Parojn's biggest problem with his diabetes is that he feels different from his friends – feelings that have only begun to set in quite recently. "At his age, he just wants to be like everyone else. For example, when there is a birthday party in school for one of his classmates, Parojn can't indulge in the cakes and Pepsis that the other kids dig into. He can only eat and

drink a little bit and, if he does, he has to compensate elsewhere, perhaps by not having any rice for the rest of the day." It is at these moments that he feels different, but his acceptance of the situation makes everything much easier to handle.

For Ratee, the most important mechanism for dealing with her son's diabetes is food control, which will in turn ensure blood glucose control. Ratee does not have to worry about food control while Parojn is at school – there is no sweet shop at the school so no temptation of sweets and soft drinks and chocolates. Instead, the school provides its students with healthy lunches. Parents are informed of the lunch menu a week ahead. Parojn knows what he can and cannot eat, and Ratee truly appreciates the peace of mind that this knowledge brings.

"I believe that people with diabetes have three different categories of food. JingJo knows about these categories and knows what to eat and what to avoid." Ratee's first category includes food Parojn cannot eat too much of or that he should avoid all together. This category includes honey, deep-fried Thai desserts, fatty foods like pork loin – which also happens to be a Thai delicacy – and other types of food high in lipids.

The second category is food that Parojn can eat in limited quantities, such as excessively sweet fruits, rice and bread.

The third category is the food group with no limitations including green vegetables and grilled fish.

"JingJo knows what types of food he can and cannot eat and he has learned what he needs to know in this area," says Ratee. "Now, we are trying to teach him about the complications that can happen if he doesn't take care of himself. We have told him a little bit, but we don't want to scare him and we don't like to tell him too much. I don't think he will comprehend it or be able to imagine that these scary things can happen to him. I am here to take care of him, so he doesn't need to be frightened with horror stories of going blind or losing a foot."

To Ratee, this is not a debatable subject. Parojn is not ready to be told of the consequences he might suffer if he ignores his diabetes. After all, his mother will protect him for as long as she can.

Natasha

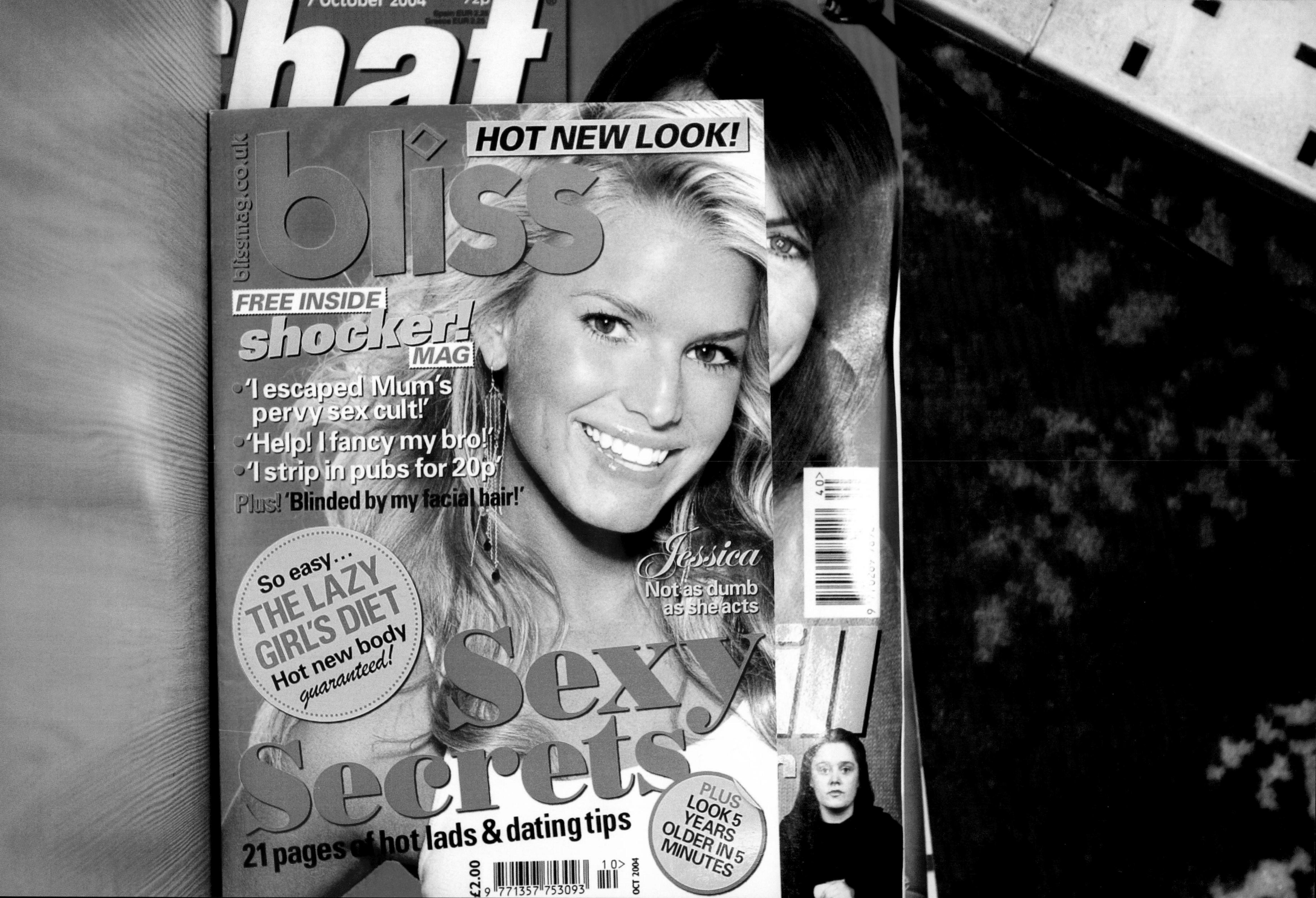

7 October 2004
chat
blissmag.co.uk
bliss
HOT NEW LOOK!
FREE INSIDE
shocker! MAG
•'I escaped Mum's pervy sex cult!'
•'Help! I fancy my bro!'
•'I strip in pubs for 20p'
Plus! 'Blinded by my facial hair!'
So easy...
THE LAZY GIRL'S DIET
Hot new body guaranteed!
Jessica
Not as dumb as she acts
Sexy Secrets
21 pages of hot lads & dating tips
PLUS LOOK 5 YEARS OLDER IN 5 MINUTES
£2.00
OCT 2004

Natasha Vye

This sixteen-year-old with the sweet and gentle smile has lived as a prisoner in her own home for two years, ever since being diagnosed with type 2 diabetes. Gradually, she uncovers a well of self-confidence and strength gurgling deep within her. She no longer wants to miss out on life. She wants to fight her diabetes and live. Natasha will make it, and when she does, she will be able to fulfil her dream of helping others who find themselves in her predicament.

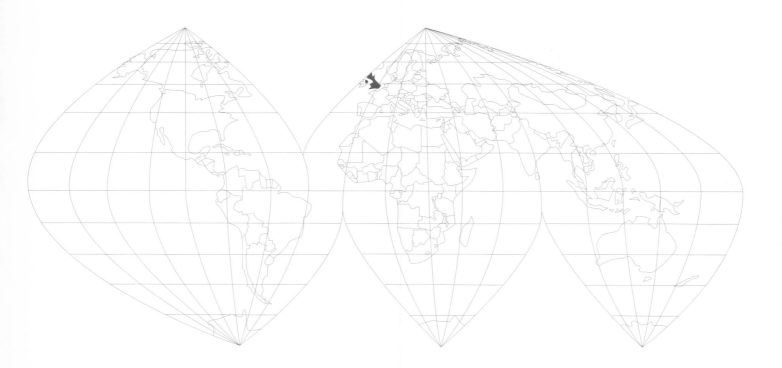

UK

In northwest Europe, between the North Sea and the Atlantic Ocean, lies England, part of the United Kingdom. The landscape is flat and rolling, with some uplands, mainly on the Scottish border. Forests cover 10 per cent of the land, while 40 per cent is suitable for grazing and 25 per cent is cultivated. The agricultural industry comprises sheep and cattle raising, and dairy farming with crop cultivation. Forestry and fishing are also very important.

The country is self-sufficient with regards to energy, due to the production of petroleum and natural gas from the reserves in the North Sea. Manufacturing of food, motor vehicles, aerospace equipment, machinery, chemicals and electronic goods accounts for over 20 per cent of the national income and relies heavily on imported raw materials. England is one of the world's financial centres, known for banking, insurance and international trade. Tourism is also a major industry, with over 18 million visitors a year.[1]

STATUS Monarchy
POPULATION 60,441,457 [2]
PEOPLE WITH DIABETES 1,700,000 [3]
LANGUAGES English, Welsh, Gaelic
RELIGIONS Protestant, Roman Catholic, Muslim, Sikh, Hindu, Jewish

[1] The country information is summarized from The Times Atlas of the World - Consice Edition, 1996.

[2] U.S. Census Bureau, International Data Base, September 30, 2004.

[3] International Diabetes Federation, 2004.

"Diabetes is getting more common in younger people, so I think they ought to start educating us."

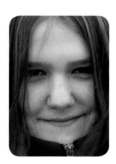

She is sitting in her math class, trying to concentrate on the blackboard that is a blur before her, when the school receptionist enters the classroom. "Your mum's coming to get you." She thinks, "Maybe my granddad has just died." Out of her mind with worry, she breaks down into tears, thinking that the dearest man in her life has passed away.

She leaves class to wait for her mother outside the school, not knowing what awaits her. When her mother gets out of the car and comes up to her, she asks, "Is it Granddad?"

"No, no, everything is fine with Granddad," says her mother, and then adds, "You're diabetic."

THE BEGINNING OF UNCERTAINTY

The diagnosis of diabetes came at the culmination of a year filled with depression and uncertainty for 16-year-old Natasha Vye.

For an entire year before her diagnosis, Natasha had felt dreadful, sinking lower and lower into a severe depression. She suffered from headaches, blurry vision, severe lethargy and thirst so extreme that she began to take large drinks to bed with her to ease night-time dehydration.

She started to stay at home from school, unable to gather the energy to get out of bed. She knew she should see a doctor, but she was afraid to learn of what might be wrong with her. Her depression drove her to expect the worst.

In November 2002, on the morning of her brother's wedding in Yorkshire, she became physically sick, vomiting just before the wedding ceremony. Later, during the reception, while gulping down huge quantities of Coke, she strangely felt better with every sip that she took.

Soon after the wedding, she agreed to go for a medical consultation, where a blood test was taken. Natasha was terrified of the results and on that day in the parking lot of her school, her mother brought her the serious news.

She remembers her mother hugging her, telling her everything would be all right. She remembers rushing home to change out of her school uniform, before leaving to go to the Children's Hospital in Bristol. She remembers not bothering to pack a bag for the hospital, seeing as the doctor had said they would only be there for a few hours.

The few hours stretched into a blur of weeks – making the memories from that time obscure.

"I don't really remember much anymore. I was in shock then. I didn't know how to react to what was happening. I've never been away from mum before, and I've never been in a hospital. When she left me at night, I cried. I kept thinking to myself, 'This is it. My life is over.'"

Natasha Vye lives in the coastal town of Clevedon, just a few miles away from Bristol. Tasha, as she is known to all, lives with her mother, Jill, and her sisters, 19-year-old Lisa, 14-year-old Jody and five-year-old Breanna. Thinking back two years to the day Natasha was diagnosed with type 2 diabetes, her mother admits, "I don't think we realised then how much our lives were going to change."

NATASHA'S STRUGGLE

//It seemed that the diabetes was controlling my life. I felt frightened and I didn't even know why."

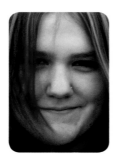

And their lives did change, especially Natasha's. She began missing days and then weeks of school, until she eventually stopped attending classes altogether and had to resort to home tutoring. Feelings of bitterness, rage and depression came over her, eating away at the little bit of self-confidence she possessed.

Natasha is a shy girl, with very low self-esteem. She attributes it to the fact that she is overweight and has been ever since the age of 10.

"I wish I could be a bit more confident. I need to have faith in myself and not be negative all the time. I was very negative in the beginning," she says. Because of her weight, doctors found it hard to classify Natasha's diabetes as either type 1 or type 2.

"They told me they didn't know and that I was in the middle," she explains. As a result, she was put on both insulin injections and tablets, before finally being diagnosed with type 2 diabetes because of her weight.

The first year was hard for the teenager. The question 'Why me?' never left Natasha's thoughts for long and she found herself going in and out of hospital.

"For the first couple of weeks, I was doing fine, my blood sugars were perfect. Then things just got harder. I don't know why. I started blaming myself. I couldn't believe I could have this diabetes thing forever. I didn't want to cope." Soon, her entire life was her small home. She did not dare venture out of the house, and saw less and less of her friends. She only wanted to be left alone. "My days were mostly just watching the telly and playing on the computer."

For Natasha, every aspect of living with diabetes is hard – but planning and diet seem to be among the most difficult.

"You just have to change your whole life: the way you do things, when you eat, what you eat, what you take with you if you go somewhere.

"And, on top of it all, I have to lose weight. I keep trying, but I just can't seem to do it. I enjoy my food! I can't say that I don't. It's hard."

Natasha also admits to disliking the idea of being the centre of attention. She believes that her introverted nature makes it even harder to deal with her diabetes, because after her diagnosis, she suddenly realised the entire family's focus was on her.

"It made me nervous – really nervous – because I'm quite shy. It seemed that the diabetes was controlling my life. I felt frightened and I didn't even know why. It felt like everything that was happening to me was so unfair."

A lot was happening to Natasha. After missing a year of school, she tried to ease back into her classes, only to find the teachers rigid and unhelpful, and the students mocking and bullying. The teachers did not understand that Natasha needed to have a drink and a snack with her at all times, even during class lectures. And her "friends" teased her about her weight and her diabetes, thinking she was using it as an excuse to miss school.

Then Natasha found herself battling another medical problem. A pilonidal sinus, a hair follicle growing backwards into the skin, was found at the base of Natasha's spine. It was very painful, regularly bleeding and causing constant discomfort. It had been there for quite some

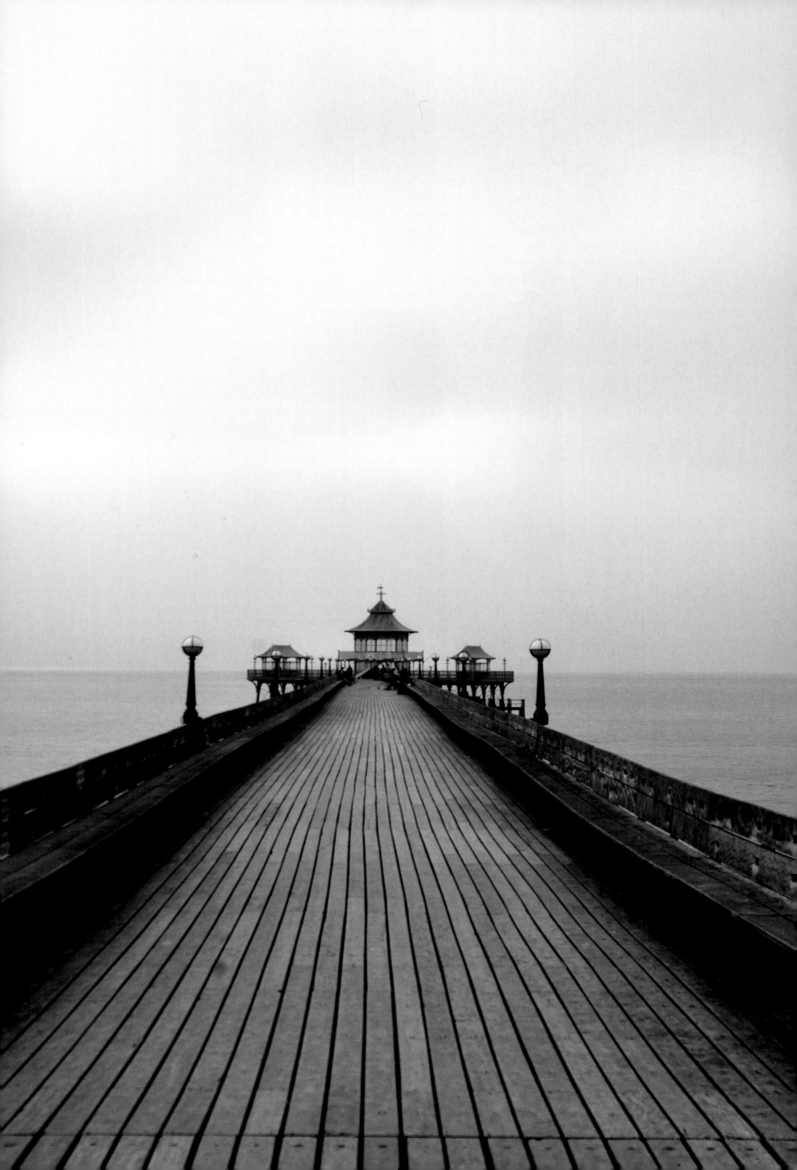

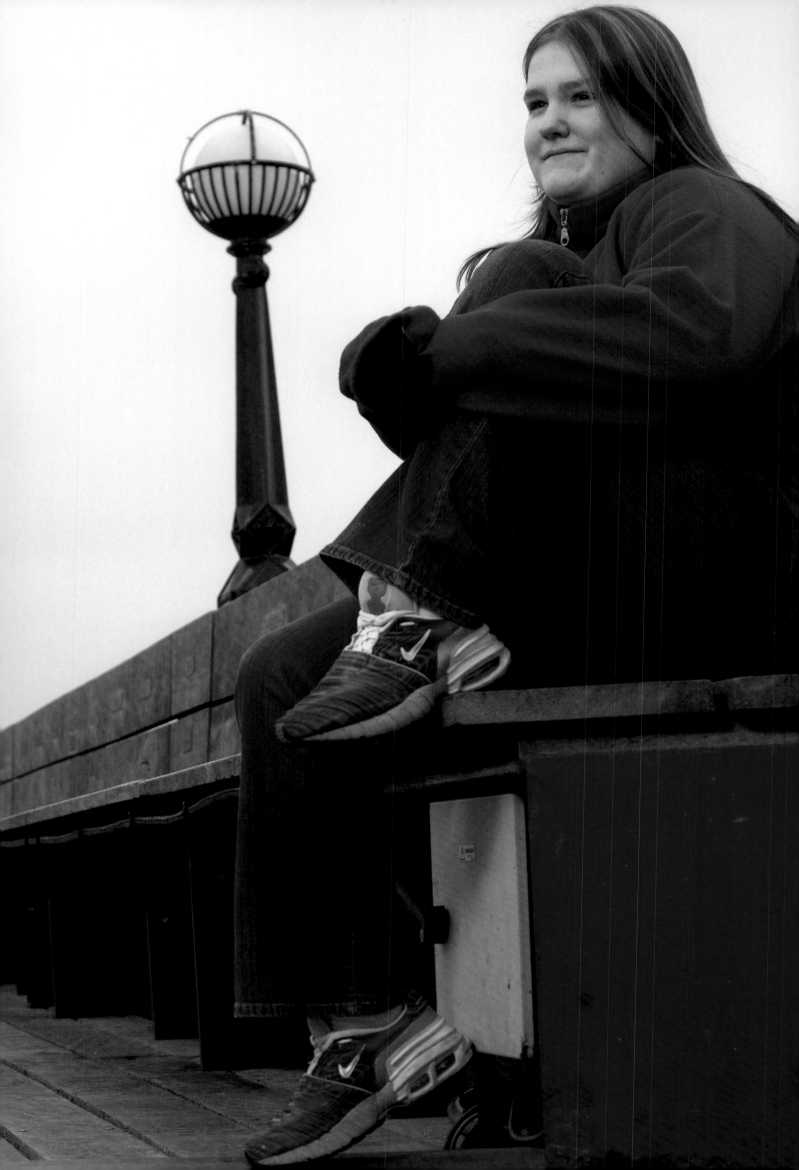

time, but Natasha had been too shy to say anything about it. When she could bare it no longer, she called her mother to have a look.

"What Tasha had was quite common, but because of the diabetes, it can cause problems," says Jill. Natasha has had to undergo three operations over the past year to remove dead and infected skin from the area, and still has one more to go. And, because of her diabetes, the delicate wound is taking a long time to heal. Therefore, strenuous exercise is out of the question, and Natasha can only stand short intervals of light physical activity before her wound begins to throb and even bleed.

Finally, about five months ago, the emotional strain became too much for Natasha. She suffered from depression and frightening panic attacks. She blamed herself and everyone around her, and she felt that she might never get her life back on track.

"It would have been good to talk to someone else about diabetes," admits Natasha. Although she and her mother went to a local diabetes event a few months ago, Natasha felt embarrassed when she found she was, by far, the youngest person with diabetes in the crowd.

"I've never talked to anyone my age that has diabetes," she says. "I just want to know that I'm not alone and that I'm not the only one with it … because sometimes, it feels that way."

A GRANDFATHER'S INFLUENCE

❚❚Granddad helped me realise that although I thought I was okay on the outside, deep inside I was trying to hide it, the anger and bitterness."

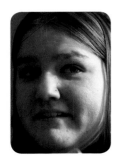

No matter how alone Natasha feels or how low her emotions sink, she can always go to her grandfather for comfort.

He is crucial to her, having been the 'father figure' in her life since her parents' seperation. Her father now has a family of his own and Natasha's relationship with him is awkward and distant.

Her grandfather, on the other hand, is very close to Natasha. "I see Granddad practically every day and he's always been there for me," she says smiling at the thought of him. "And, I've always been the special one to him. He gives us kids his time, and although he has prostate cancer, he doesn't waste time worrying about that. He cares about us instead and makes sure we're well looked after. It's enough that he's always there when I need him."

Natasha has needed him many times over the past two years – but never more than when she almost gave up her will to live. At that point, she simply refused to take her insulin.

"It was a build-up, really, and had been for ages and it just came out of me – I just don't know what happened," says Natasha. "I wanted to die. I didn't want to go on with the problems piling up on me, one after the other."

Jill shudders at the memory. "You can imagine what that was like for me! I knew she was up there, in her room, refusing to take her insulin," she recalls. "I had to call her Granddad to talk to her."

Natasha remembers the defining moment when her grandfather helped her break away from her misery:

"Granddad came and sat upstairs on my bed, and we had a good talk and a good cry, and I felt guilty because I made him cry and upset him," she says. "I didn't want to ever do that again.

"Granddad helped me realise that although I thought I was okay on the outside, deep inside I was trying to hide it, all the anger and bitterness. And then it all just came out one day and I just didn't want to go on. But he was there for me when I couldn't go to my mum. I'd already dumped enough problems on her, and I thought that I wanted to be alone."

Natasha finally realised the futility of what she was doing. With the help of her grandfather and mother, she decided to put an end to the destruction she was causing herself.

"I said to myself, 'Stop being so stupid,' and I promised

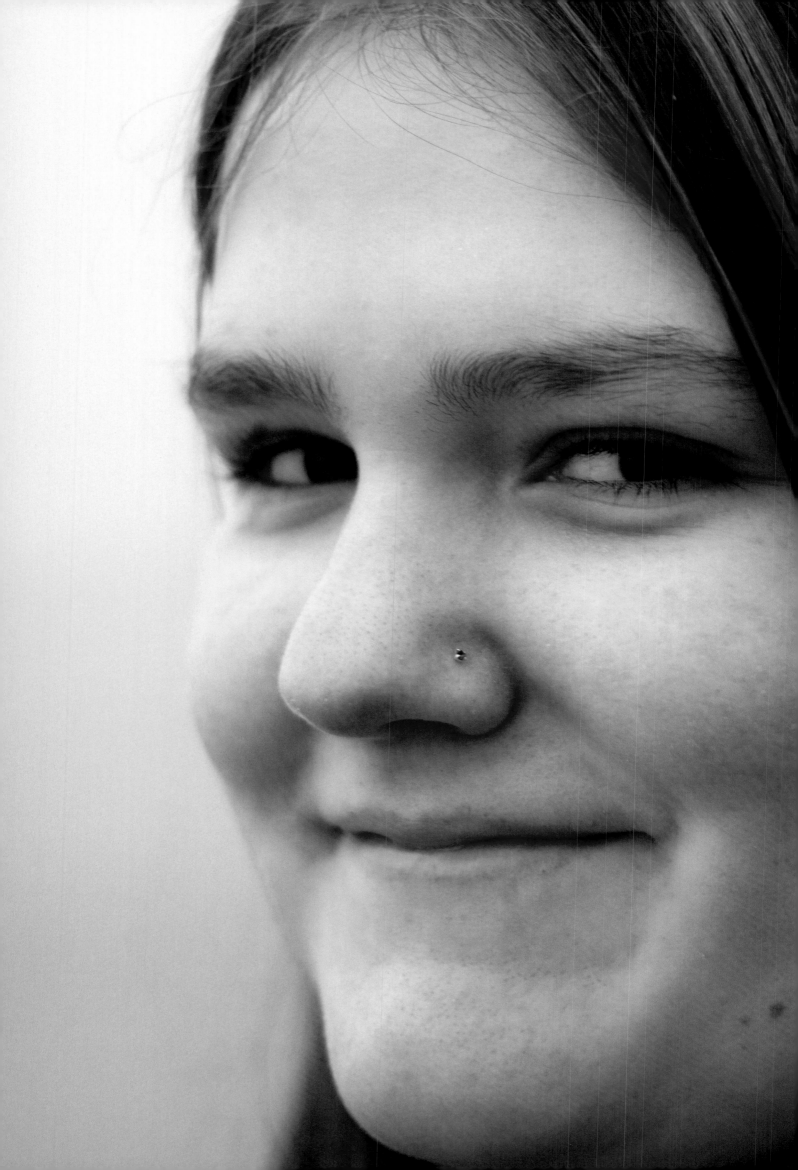

myself I'd never do that to myself again. I think of Mum and Granddad and I reckon I don't want to put any more strain on him because it'll kill him. I don't want that."

REGAINING LOST CONFIDENCE

▮▮I thought I was going to stick out like a sore thumb and everyone would be staring at me."

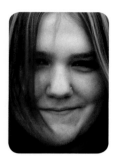

Gradually and with the help of several outside factors, Natasha is beginning to find the strength to go on. She is trying to see more of her friends, going out with them to cafés after school, and hanging out with them during the evenings.

Slowly, she is also being integrated back into school by attending classes three days a week, while continuing with home tutoring. The experience of going back to school is not as daunting as she once feared it would be.

In fact, many things are becoming easier for her. For example, a few months ago, she went away for three weeks to visit her married brother in Germany and spend some time with his family. The independence she gained from those three weeks gave her confidence a strong boost and she realised that being part of the outside world was not as scary as she once thought it would be.

"I used to hate going out in the street. I felt everyone would stare at me and say, 'Oh, look at the fat, ugly thing walking,' or something like that. And I had a fear of people watching me eat. I just used to think that everyone knew that I was diabetic and I was embarrassed about it. I don't feel that way anymore. I've realised there's nothing to be embarrassed about."

Her love of music has also helped her.

"I just love Blink 182, I'm obsessed with them!" Natasha gushes like the teenager she is whenever she speaks of her favourite boy band. "I love their music. I just can't explain it; I feel great when I listen to them."

Very recently, Natasha, her sister Jody and one of their friends attended a Blink 182 concert in Cardiff, not far from where they live. "That concert was a big step for me, because it was the first time I was around so many people. It's something I've always wanted to do. But I kept changing my mind a million times about going – I was frightened.

"I thought I was going to stick out like a sore thumb and everyone would stare at me. But I didn't! I was wearing jeans and a black top, and I fit in quite well! It felt great being in the middle of all those people! My confidence has gone up so much since that, and I'd do it all over again."

Natasha danced all night, jumping around with the thousands of other fans. She is finally beginning to understand that she can do anything a "normal" person can do, and she admits that there is no reason why diabetes should hold her back.

LEARNING TO LIVE WITH DIABETES

▮▮I wish I could go back in time and change my lifestyle. When I wasn't feeling well, I had the suspicion that I would have diabetes, because I knew a little bit about it but not much."

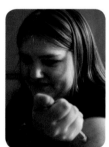

Natasha still, although rarely, has some emotionally difficult days, when she cannot help but feel angry, miserable and sorry for herself.

"But then I remind myself that I could be really worse off – with cancer or something – and that I should get my act together, I guess."

Natasha lets her long, straight hair with the pink highlights, dyed especially for the Blink 182 concert, fall in front of her face so she can hide behind it.

"I wish I could go back in time and change my lifestyle. When I wasn't feeling well, I had the suspicion that I would have diabetes, because I knew a little bit about it but not much." Diabetes is in Natasha's family; her grandmother had diabetes, and Natasha can't help but worry about the complications that she too may one day face.

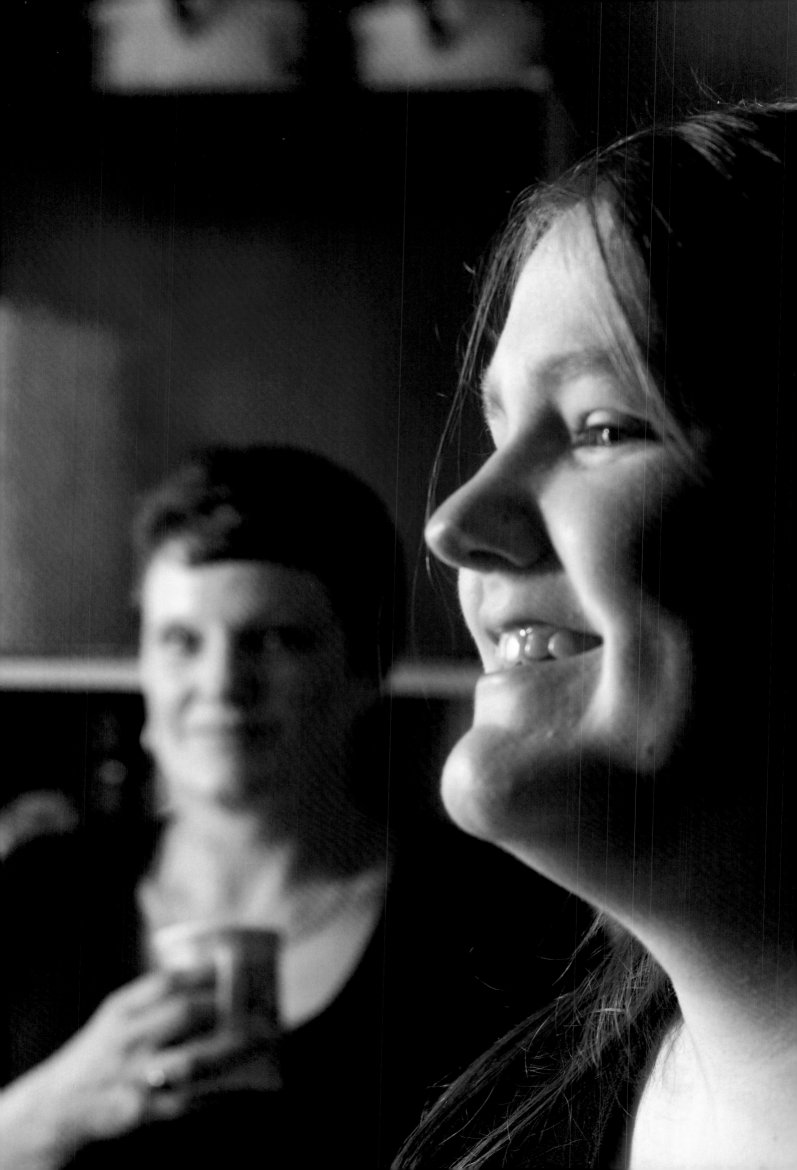

"I know now that you have to get to the point where you control the diabetes and it doesn't control you anymore. I'm not as down on myself as I was before. I'm a little more positive. I go out a lot more and see my friends, whereas I never used to go out before. I feel normal again now. I used to feel useless, diseased, a walking mound of fat. I'm more in control of myself now. Maybe because I'm getting older and I realise stuff I didn't realise before, like, I've got to eat healthy and take my insulin, even if I am having a bad day."

Natasha picks at the black Blink 182 wristband on her left hand and admits that she has been missing out on life. All she wants now is to live her life to the fullest and no longer be the kind of person that stays inside, afraid. Although she once allowed diabetes to stand in her way and stop her from accomplishing all that she wanted to be, she now knows it can no longer do that.

"Everyone said to me that things will get better. And I feel it now. It's becoming easier to handle. It was a big deal at first but now it's just something I've got to live with. I'm used to it now. I still feel like I'm learning but that's OK." Natasha feels that right now she must get her eating habits in order and stop worrying so much. "I worry a lot, and I think that's why I get so nervous. I worry about the future and what might happen next. I worry that I could get like a kidney infection or something like that, due to the diabetes. I am taking care of myself but sometimes I let myself go a bit and I have to control that."

Nowadays, Natasha makes an effort to get out of the house. She goes on walks with her mother to browse around the nearby shops and warm up with a cup of tea. In the afternoons, she sees as much of her friends as she can, walking to meet them, so she gets some exercise. Her concern now is to lose her excess weight and she knows she must start making more healthy food choices if she wants to accomplish that goal.

"I've been to a dietician once, and it just didn't help me. I think my problem is that I eat between meals and, except for walking, I don't get much exercise. I resort to comfort eating," confesses Natasha, who loves pizzas and Indian curry, and dislikes fruits and vegetables. "I need to change my diet and eat more healthily. I know that!"

HOPES FOR THE FUTURE

❚❚I want to be a midwife. I just think it must be such a rewarding job and I adore babies."

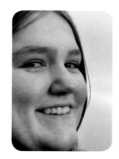

"I am proud of my daughter," says Jill. "She has coped brilliantly with her condition, even though at times it has been extremely hard and unfair for her. We have been through all the emotions: bitterness, anger, wishing she were dead. But I think we are, at last, seeing light at the end of the tunnel."

Natasha and her mother are living through Natasha's diabetes day by day, learning from the gruelling start and knowing they can rely on one another for strength. Although Jill can sometimes be a bit overprotective of Natasha, as well as of all her children, Natasha does not resent any of it.

"Mum worries constantly, but she wouldn't be a mum if she didn't worry! She's been great. She's always there to look after me and give me advice. We've always been close, but diabetes brought us even closer. So I did get something good out of it!"

Jill has learned to stop blaming herself for her daughter's condition, and instead works at making sure her other daughters live healthy lifestyles that will prevent them from getting type 2 diabetes.

"Everyone in the family now checks their blood glucose levels regularly, just to be on the safe side. Sometimes I worry of course, that Breanna is too thin or one of the girls is eating too much junk food. But I look out for all of them and make sure they look out for themselves as well," says Jill.

Natasha is learning to take better care of herself and even has hopes for the future. She dreams of working at a part-time job, admitting that she would love some extra pocket money, as well as the chance to get out more often and meet more people. "I've never had the confidence to get a job before, but maybe now that will change."

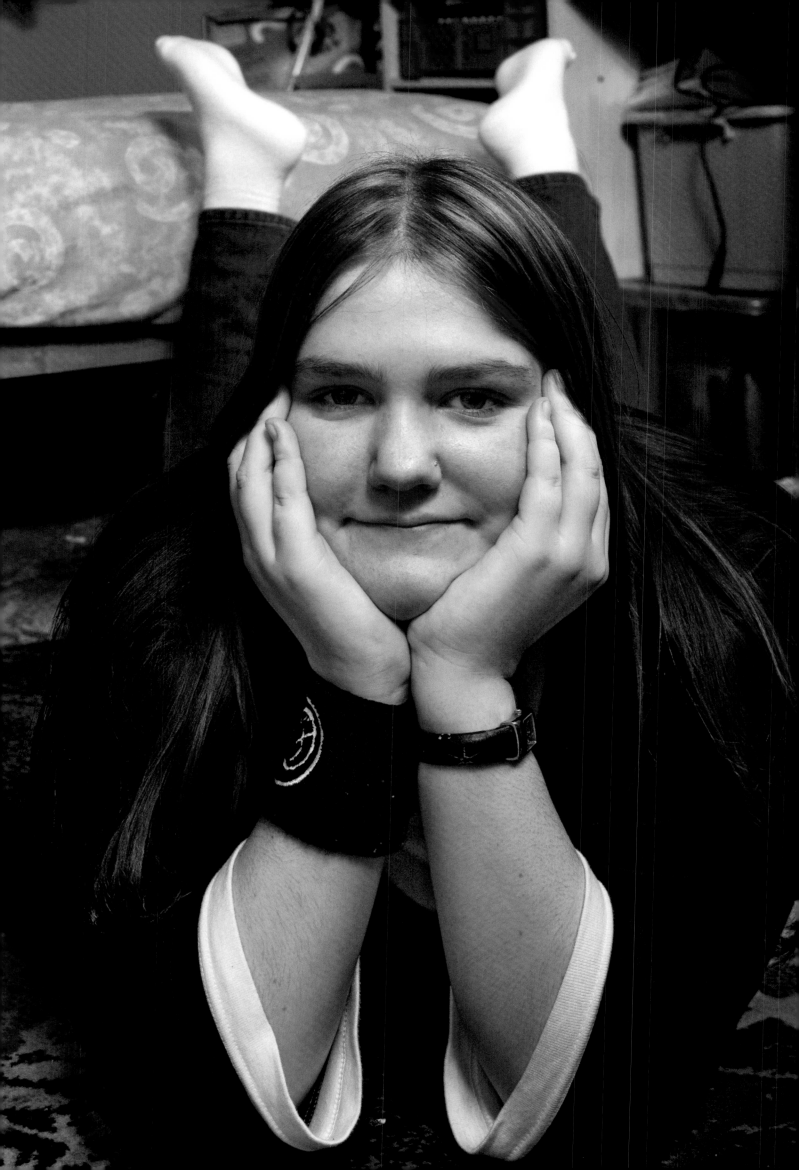

Meanwhile, she is working hard at catching up with the rest of her classmates at school. The table in the warm and cosy kitchen where she takes her home tutoring classes has a small pile of books on it. On the top of the pile is Natasha's *Health and Social Care* book, the title of which happens to be her favourite subject.

"I want to be a midwife. I just think it must be such a rewarding job and I adore babies," admits Natasha, describing herself as the maternal type. She became very close to her little nephew, 18-month-old Jamie, while she was on her trip to Germany.

"I can't talk to him on the phone, Hearing his voice makes me cry so much! I love him to bits, he's so cute, and I miss him terribly."

Pictures of little Jamie, as well as countless other family members, are all over the house. And although Natasha knows she must get out more often, which is something she wants, she admits that she is a homebody at heart.

"I like being on my own and I like where we live. It's quiet, and not so crowded like Bristol, so I want my future to be here. I'm laid back and quiet, so it's perfect for me."

What Natasha's future does not include are moments of irresponsible behaviour. During her bouts of depression and anger, Natasha smoked, drank and hung out with the "wrong" crowd.

"I don't know what I was thinking," she says. "Maybe I was seeking attention – a different sort of attention than what I was getting. Maybe I was crying out for help. But I wanted to hurt myself even more than I was already hurting, and I was feeling self-destructive. Mum was there for me though, as was Granddad, and I swore I would never do something like that again. I felt terrible and sick; my blood sugar levels were so high whenever I started drinking and I hated the feeling."

Jill had no choice but to ground her daughter when she noticed the rebellious behaviour and, luckily, the firm hand taught Natasha a lesson. For her, the future means taking care of herself. Harming herself is no longer an option. She wants to live.

A DESIRE TO HELP

"I think everyone should know about diabetes and know how to take care of themselves."

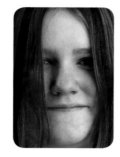

"Tasha would bend over backwards to help young people become more aware of the risk of diabetes, so that they wouldn't have to suffer and go through what she has gone through," says Jill, proudly.

Natasha has noticed that at her school, none of the students are taught anything about diabetes, or the risk factors that can lead to a diagnosis of type 2.

"Diabetes is getting more common in younger people, so I think they ought to start educating us," says Natasha. "You have to become more aware and learn what to look for."

Perhaps by exercising regularly and making healthy food choices, Natasha could have avoided diabetes, but that possibility is something she wishes she had known about a long time ago.

"If I had known that I was at risk of getting diabetes because of my lifestyle, I would have done something about my weight and not carried on like I was. There were times I would go baking with my friends, and we'd eat an entire tin of chocolate frosting. That was just stupid! I should never have done things like that!"

Gradually, Natasha is finding ways to help others learn from her experience. During her latest surgery on the infected hair follicle, she permitted the surgical team to take a sample of tissue from her wound to help benefit diabetes research. Moreover, she has talked to several medical students about her experiences and life with diabetes.

"Mum thought I should talk to them to build up my confidence," says Natasha. "But more than that, I want to help raise awareness. I think everyone should know about diabetes and know how to take care of themselves, so they don't ever get diabetes. If there is some way I can help people realise that, then I will do it. Maybe that way, I can help myself."

Deeb

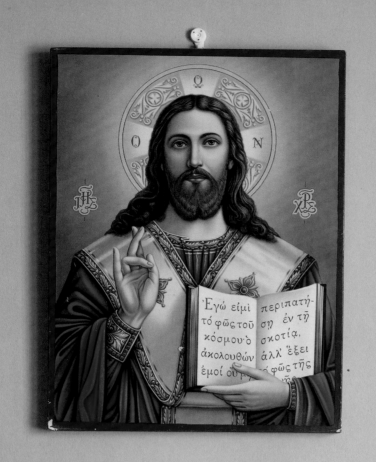

Ἐγώ εἰμι περιπατή-
τό φῶς τοῦ ση ἐν τῇ
κόσμου· ὁ σκοτία,
ἀκολουθῶν ἀλλ᾽ ἕξει
ἐμοί ου μ· τό φῶς τῆς

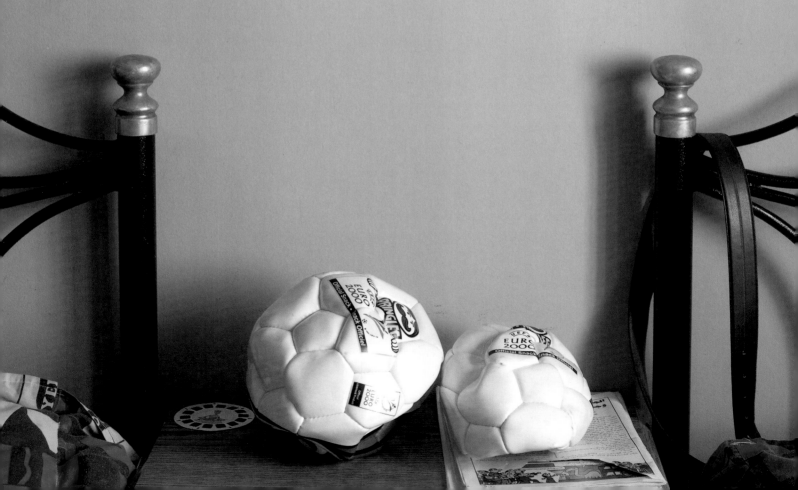

Deeb Kameel Ghnnma

Deeb, a young man struggling to accept his diagnosis of type 2 diabetes, prays every day for the strength and resolve to fight and control the diabetes, believing with all his heart that his faith will step in and rescue him. Yet deep down inside, beneath the feelings of fulfilment, serenity and hope that surge through prayer, Deeb knows that the necessary transformation can only come from within him.

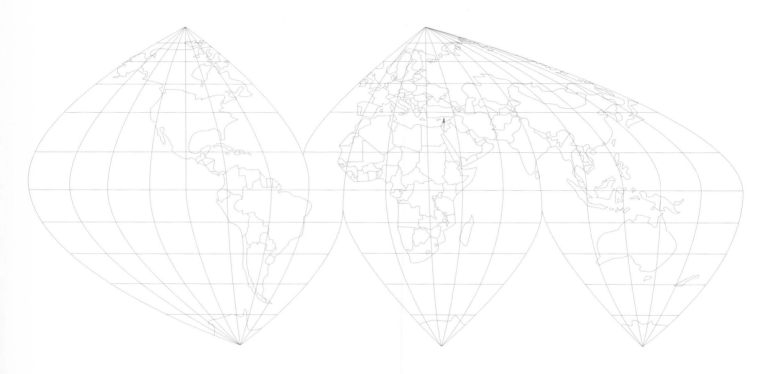

JORDAN

Situated in southwest Asia, Jordan is bordered by Syria to the north, Iraq and Saudi Arabia to the east and Israel to the west. The central spine of the country is highland plateaus and hilly regions that run from north to south, with a short coastline to the south known as the Gulf of Aqaba. In the west lies the world's lowest point at more than 400 metres below sea level: the Dead Sea. The eastern desert area is a semi-arid steppe which receives little rainfall. Most people live in the northwest corner of the country where the climate is cooler and moister.

Jordan's economy is mostly based on tourism, workers' remittance and foreign aid. Pharmaceuticals, fertilisers, potassium, phosphates, fruits and vegetables are the main exports.[1]

STATUS Monarchy

POPULATION 5,759,732 [2]

PEOPLE WITH DIABETES 300,000 [3]

LANGUAGES Arabic, English

RELIGIONS Sunni Muslim, Christian, Shia Muslim

[1] The country information is summarized from The Times Atlas of the World - Consice Edition, 1996.

[2] U.S. Census Bureau, International Data Base, September 30, 2004.

[3] Jordanian Society for the Care of Diabetes, 2004.

"It's easy to forget yourself if you have type 2 diabetes."

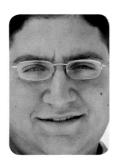

He hurries in, his head bowed in respect, and finds a seat towards the front, at the far end of the wooden pew. He focuses his attention on the young man leading the youthful congregation. An intense expression of acceptance and belonging settles amongst his features as he straightens and prepares to sing a hymn. It is at moments like these, when attending church or congregating with his religious youth group, that he feels complete.

Deeb Kameel Ghnnma is a devoutly religious young man of 22. His faith is a constant companion, both in difficult times and joyful moments. Without his strong faith, Deeb would not have been able to deal with his diagnosis of type 2 diabetes. As it is, Deeb attributes his diagnosis to God's will.

"At first, I experienced moments of anger, confusion and hurt. I didn't really understand what it meant to have diabetes; I assumed I was now paying for my love of sugar and everything sweet. But I truly believe this is all part of God's plan; the plan he has for all of us. That's why I have this sense of acceptance. God chose me to go through this for a reason. God thinks I will be strong enough to overcome it. Now I just have to find the strength!"

Deeb is fully aware that he has not yet achieved the strength or the ability to control his diabetes and learn how to live with it correctly. He knows the importance of committing to an exercise plan and a healthy diet, and yet his resolve repeatedly vanishes at the slightest temptation. He was diagnosed in November 2002, when he was in his second year of university. At the time, he weighed 145 kilos. His current weight is 127 kilos, but he knows there is still a long way to go.

"The problem is that I don't feel sick; I don't feel anything. It's easy to forget yourself if you have type 2 diabetes. That's the problem with diabetes. It's a disease that's like a double-edged sword. If you know how to deal with it, then you're okay. If you don't, then it's as dangerous as cancer."

GENETIC DISPOSITION

His shock was almost physical in its strength, and he immediately scheduled an appointment with his doctor.

Deeb is Kameel's and Aida's eldest child, followed by 19-year-old Zeina and seven-year-old Zeid. The close-knit family live in Amman, Jordan's ever-growing capital, in a moderate-sized apartment built by Deeb's engineer father, Kameel, who also has type 2 diabetes. Kameel learned of his diabetes in early 2001, almost two years before Deeb was diagnosed.

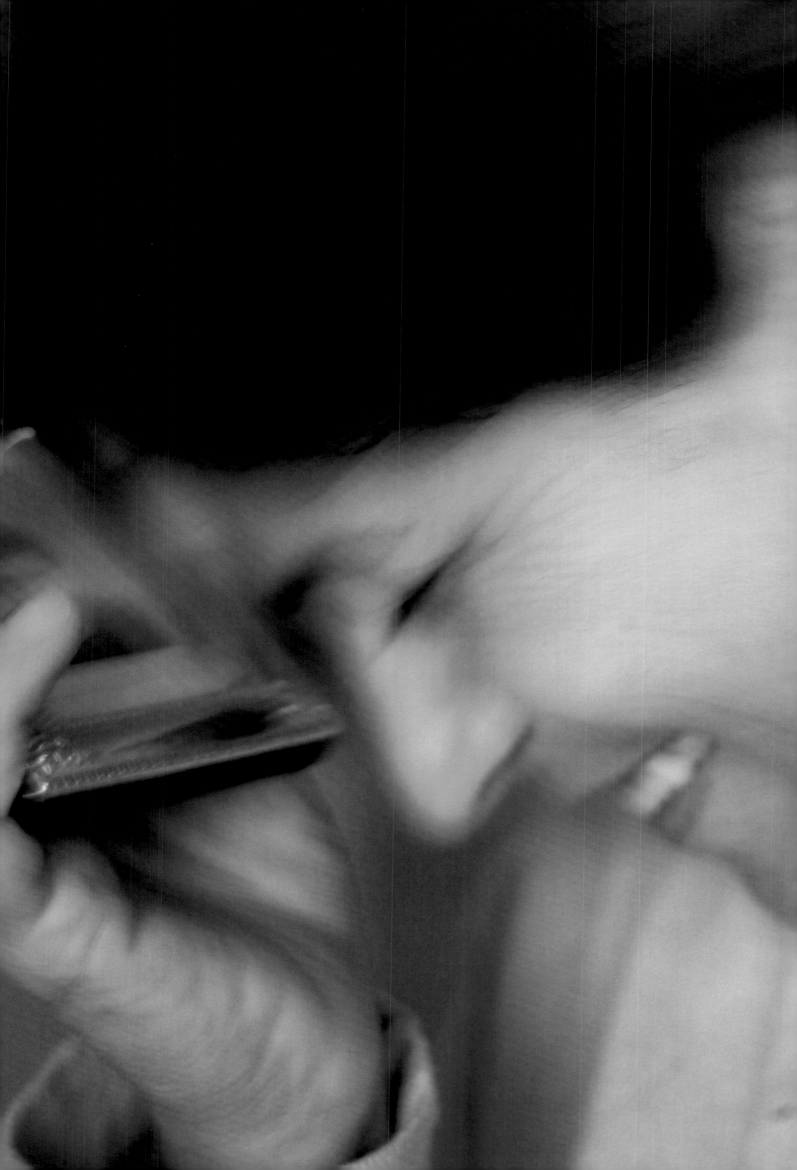

Before learning of his diabetes, Kameel had always been in the habit of testing his blood sugar levels regularly, aware of the family history of diabetes. Relatives on both his father's and mother's sides have been diagnosed with diabetes.

During a visit to his sister's home, Kameel decided to bring out the glucometer, knowing he had been feeling out of sorts all day, and for a few days back as well. Less than two months earlier, he had been suffering from an enormous personal problem that he refuses to talk about to this day. Even at the time of this conflict he shared his burden with no one, choosing to let it fester within him, suffering sleepless nights and bouts of panic. He is convinced that the stress induced by this hidden anguish is what led to his diabetes, because that day Kameel's blood sugar level was very high and extremely dangerous. His shock was almost physical in its strength, and he immediately scheduled an appointment with his doctor.

A MOTHER'S INTUITION

❚❚Something told me to get that glucometer and test his blood; like someone had just whispered the idea into my ear."

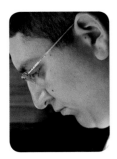

Kameel's diagnosis did not automatically mean the rest of the family would have to succumb to regular testing of their blood sugar levels. Aida made sure Deeb and his sister Zeina tested their blood glucose every once in a while, but she never expected an unusual reading. Her son Deeb was undoubtedly overweight, but active and energetic. To Aida, Deeb was too young to suffer from a disorder like type 2 diabetes, nicknamed the 'old man's disease' in Jordan.

Her peace of mind, however, was short-lived. During the last days of October 2002, something spoke to Aida and told her to test Deeb's blood sugar level. "We were watching TV, and Deeb got up to fetch himself some water from the kitchen," says Aida, remembering a not-so-distant past, her eyes reflecting a pain only she can understand.

"Something told me to get that glucometer and test his blood; like someone had just whispered the idea into my ear. Maybe it was because Kameel's struggle was constantly on my mind. Whatever it was, I thank God every day for opening our eyes."

She stares down at her hands, her voice losing its urgency but retaining its pain. "When I saw that his blood sugar level was so high, I didn't know how to react," says Aida in a voice devoid of all emotion. She was too shocked to take in what Deeb was trying to tell her; he had just eaten, and he had had a lot of sweets and chocolates that day. His excuses were washing over her, but she barely registered them as she refused to believe her teenage son had type 2 diabetes. She immediately scheduled an appointment with the doctor, dreading the outcome. Deeb underwent some tests, and soon after the family's fears were confirmed. "He had diabetes. And the main reason was his weight."

Living with uncontrolled diabetes and unregulated blood sugar levels can lead to a horrific list of complications. Aida fears Deeb may lose his eyesight, suffer a heart attack, or end up with kidney failure. She knows that hypertension – high blood pressure – can accompany diabetes, and she knows that diabetes affects small blood vessels, which may lead to limb amputations. Therefore, she thinks she has every right to fear for her son.

"Deeb just walks into the room, sees me crying and wonders why I am so upset," says Aida. "He thinks I am making a big deal out of nothing. Oh God, when will he understand?"

Aida's eyes shine with unshed tears as she speaks of what she describes as the 'deepest emotional pain' of her life. Aida feels that Deeb pays no heed to the seriousness of his condition. He shows no fear or worry, and gives the impression that he does not understand the magnitude of what may happen if he fails to lose weight and does not learn to control his diabetes. Aida admits haltingly that she has spent many a dark night huddled on the couch, trying to contain the tears of worry and frustration coursing down her face, as she prays to God to help her son face this obstacle and overcome it.

DEEB'S DRIVE AND DEVOTION

❚❚ I have too much faith in God to allow myself to worry or be fearful. I know I will overcome this."

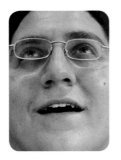

Deeb, nicknamed 'Deebo' by his family and friends, is a young man living a full, normal life – his interests are varied and his free time is always packed. His lovable nature and his social, outgoing character enable him to be himself, confidently and self-assuredly, among his many friends. Watching soccer games, smoking flavoured-tobacco water pipes on the roof and sauntering the halls of the local mall are all activities he enjoys regularly with his friends, but his primary interest lies elsewhere.

For Deeb, religion is his driving force; he attends church regularly and is a member of two different religious youth groups. His Bible is a constant companion, its cover worn from years of tender handling. He spends a lot of time in his room listening to religious songs and reading his Bible.

"I love reading the Sacred Book, praying in my room, trying to find spiritual healing. It makes me feel instantly better."

He also reads many other things. He recently finished both an Arabic translation of *Men are from Venus, Women are from Mars* and a book entitled *And God Said*, which ties the Bible to science and explains, through strong scientific proof, that concepts like the Big Bang theory and Darwin's theory of the evolution of the species are just that: only theories and not fact.

Deeb can definitely boast a full life; so full, in fact, that diabetes seems to rank low on his list of priorities. "God helps me with the diabetes and with everything else. But still, I sometimes forget about it," he says.

Deeb explains that he overlooks his diabetes because he doesn't feel it physically; he has reiterated repeatedly that he feels neither sick nor ill. He does, however, feel his obesity, quickly losing his breath after climbing a short flight of stairs in his church or bouncing a soccer ball on his knee in his bedroom. He has heard diabetes described as the 'silent killer,' and he knows it is because diabetes becomes dangerous when it is ignored and complications begin to set in. He simply chooses to forget every now and then.

Deeb dons an expression of indifference to mask his hurt and embarrassment as he describes how his weight, and not his diabetes, is the rampant subject in his parents' arguments with him. "I sometimes feel suffocated by my mom and dad, and I wish they would stop bringing up my weight all the time and leave me alone to deal with it. It's not true that I'm not at all afraid, which is what they think," says Deeb.

"I have too much faith in God to allow myself to worry or be fearful. I know I will overcome this. Sometimes, deep down, I do get a bit afraid when I think of all the complications that come from diabetes. I don't want to become blind or lose a foot or any of all those other things that can happen, God forbid. But look, I don't eat out of a fear or because of some emotional problem. I just eat because I like to eat! I enjoy it!"

Deeb suspects his desire for sugar has increased since his diagnosis; that is his explanation for his uncontrollable sweet tooth. He has always liked soft drinks and chocolate bars and chips and fast food burgers; the list of 'favourite foods' is endless. Deeb knows that these foods should be avoided by someone with type 2 diabetes and he does feel that he has begun to cut down.

"I want to live my life without even the tiniest hint of worry. I do," he says vehemently. "Right now, all I can do is pray for the strength that will help me through this."

In terms of physical activity, Deeb has been in and out of a few gyms, inconsistent in his attendance and unable to find the right training program for himself. Today, he walks and plays soccer to make sure he gets sufficient exercise.

Physical activity is crucial in Deeb's case, as dieting alone will only be tedious work with slow and barely discernible results. Deeb currently loses his breath after a few minutes

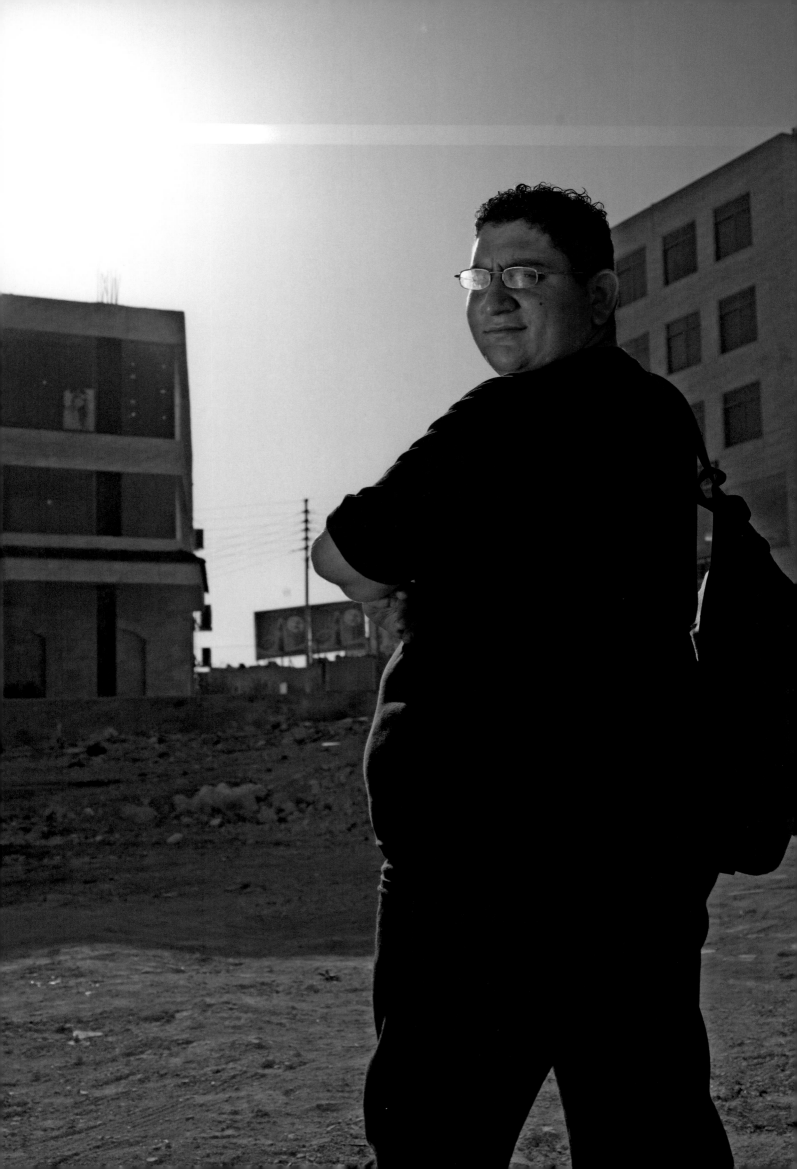

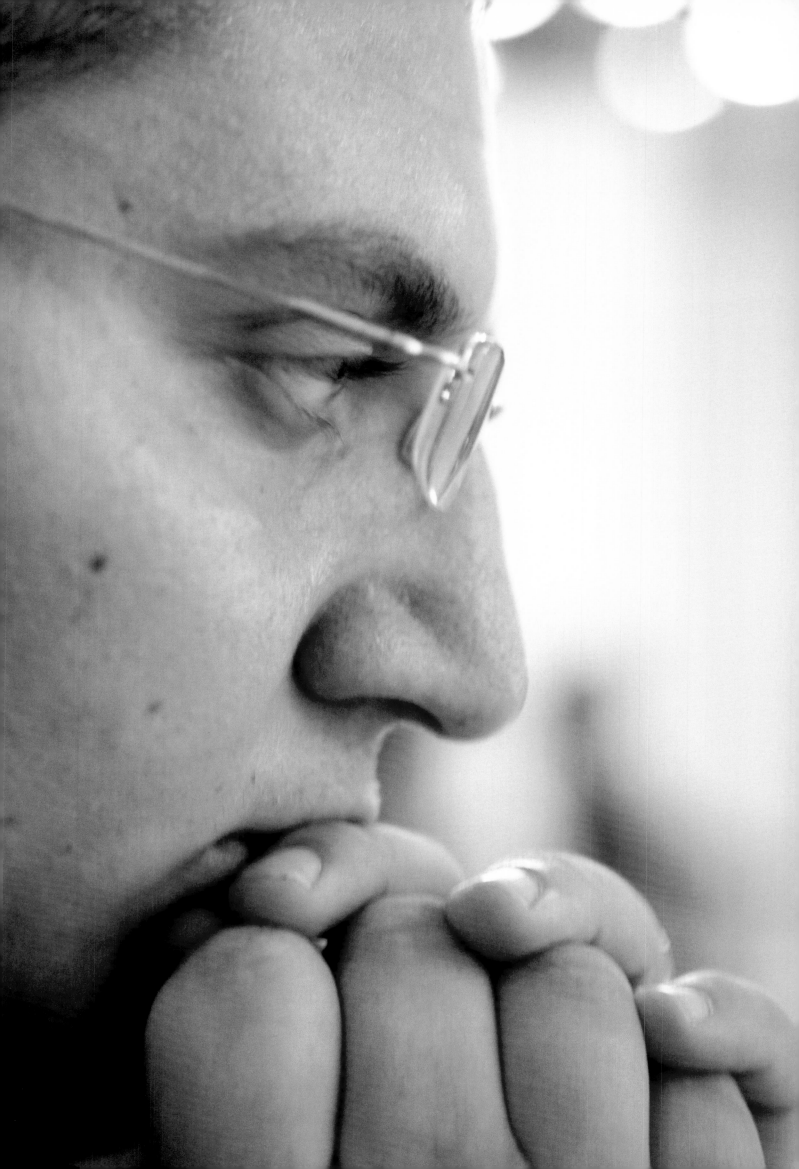

of light exercise, but with a little effort he will eventually become more fit.

"I've lost 18 kilos since I was first diagnosed over two years ago, and I definitely feel better after having lost the weight," says Deeb. "I have a better temperament; I feel faster and fitter. I guess I'll just improve if I continue to lose weight."

Deeb takes a deep breath and attempts to explain how he is indeed beginning to take his disease more seriously. "I don't think I am in denial. I check my blood sugar regularly: every Saturday morning as soon as I wake up. I've stopped hiding my diabetes like it's something I should be ashamed of, and instead I talk about it to my friends. They know I have diabetes now, which is a great help. If one of them catches me with a can of Pepsi, they make sure I throw it away. Their encouragement is appreciated. So is my parents'. I just wish it wasn't so constant!"

PEER PRESSURE

❚❚Sometimes I feel like I don't want to graduate; I meet a new batch of freshmen every year and I love it!"

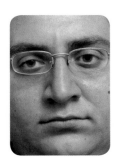

Both Deeb and his family admit to his inability to say 'no' to his peers. When the youths of his church group decide to go out for a late dinner at one of the fast food joints after a religious meeting, he can't help but accompany them.

"I'm a pushover," jokes Deeb, his delightful sense of humour apparent in everything he says or does. His numerous friends mean a lot to him. Currently a fourth-year student majoring in mechatronics[1] at Hashemite University, Deeb spent his first three years of college making as many friends and acquaintances on campus as possible. He used to skip classes often, so he would have the chance to spend time with various groups of friends.

"Sometimes I feel like I don't want to graduate; I meet a new batch of freshmen every year and I love it! We

call the freshmen students 'Smurfs' here in Jordan." Deeb laughs, then gives a shrug and a smile. "I have to buckle down though; I want to graduate by 2006. Then hopefully I'll get my Master's degree, and teach here at my university. That way, I'll still be hanging around for a while!"

Deeb's friends play an important role in his life, but none of them have diabetes, and none of them can truly understand the seriousness of Deeb's condition. He does not know of others of his age with diabetes, but he has a friend who was diagnosed with cancer and is constantly in and out of hospitals. As Deeb speaks of this friend, his playful nature departs for a moment.

"My friend was in hospital for an entire six months once; he was doing really badly at that point. But with the grace of God, he's recovered, and he's doing so much better now. He's attending classes at the university, working towards his degree, living a normal life and happy to be alive. This encouraged me so much, I felt so filled with hope. At that point, I could almost see God's touch on my friend's spirit. My friend found the strength to fight." He pauses, and his gaze shifts upwards. "I can find it too."

SOCIAL OBLIGATIONS

❚❚...Telling him not to eat this or that, embarrassing him in public. I wish I had never done that."

The high prevalence of diabetes in the Middle Eastern region might be attributed to special social and cultural traits that Deeb's family embodies. A huge percentage of the population smoke, either to deal with stressful living conditions or to be 'part of the crowd'. Social functions are the main form of entertainment in the region, and food is always served at any type of gathering. Arabs are generous souls, quick to throw open their doors in welcome and offering any guest a steady stream of food and drink in enticement, oblivious of that guest's medical restrictions.

"As Arabs, our social events are gatherings with friends and family to share food," says Aida. "We had a very social life. People were always inviting us over and we

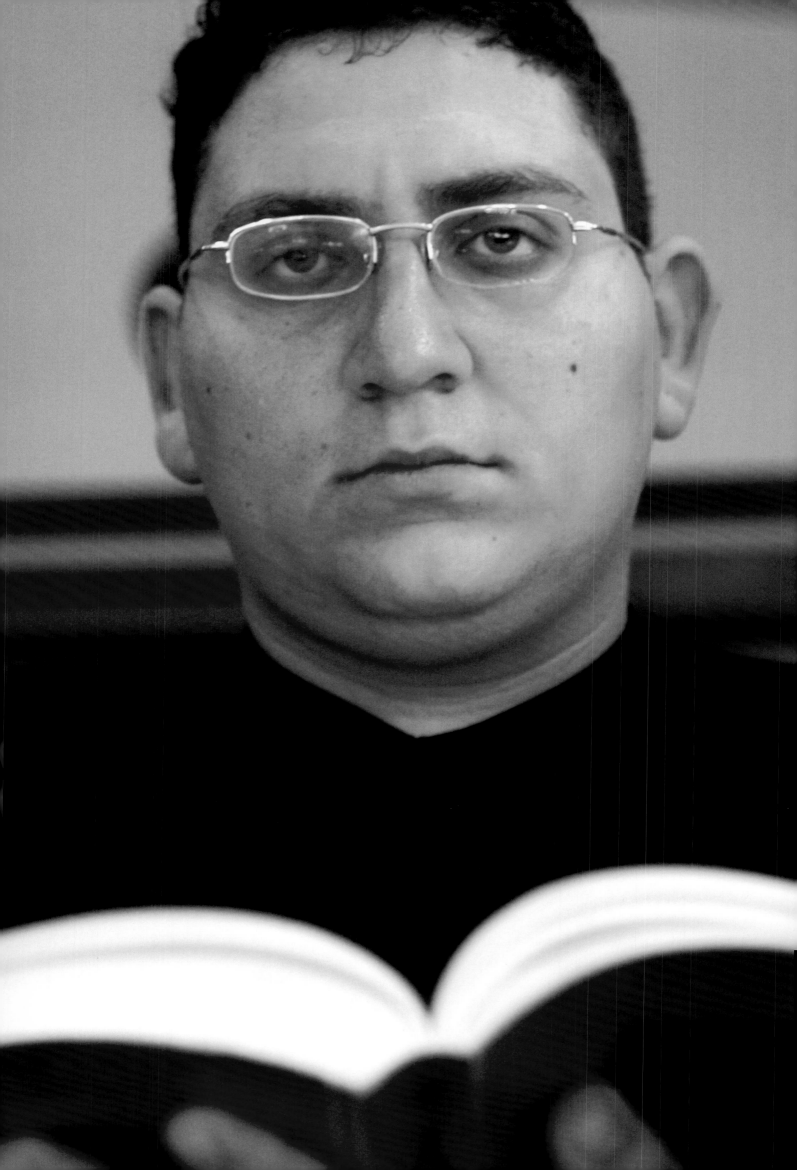

were always returning the invitation, and there was food everywhere. I would sometimes admonish Deebo, giving him smaller portions than his siblings and cousins, telling him not to eat this or that, embarrassing him in public. I wish I had never done that. I should never have made such a big deal out of it. But I didn't know what else to do! People here can't mind their own business; grown adults would comment on my little boy's weight and tease him. They meant no harm, but the harm was done."

Deeb has had to learn to say no whenever he is offered a Christmas treat while visiting friends and relatives during the holidays. He still succumbs sometimes, but he has recently vowed to stick to his resolve to lose weight. Deeb's mother has changed her style of cooking, eliminating the ghee – a butter-like substance used in Middle Eastern cooking – and introducing a wider variety of vegetables and salads in their meals. Nevertheless, Aida still has to buy a small pack of the special butter every now and then, whenever she has a lunch or dinner party and knows she will be cooking for guests.

FAMILIAL CONCERN – FOR DEEB AND FROM DEEB

❙❙I blame myself, I do. We shouldn't have made his weight such an issue. When he began gaining weight, we all made such a big fuss of our beautiful, healthy, chubby baby boy."

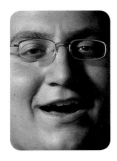

When the family sits down for lunch, which is the main meal of the day in Jordan, Aida serves the food, placing reasonable portions on each plate. She tries to ensure that the dishes centre more on proteins and vegetables than on carbohydrates and starches. White bread has been substituted with whole wheat bread in the Ghnnma household, and vegetable soup is a weekly occurrence on the family's dining table. The rest is up to Deeb; he must find the strength to lose weight and exercise.

Deeb's family want to reach the point where Deeb wants to treat himself well. Instead of walking down the right path in order to please his mother or his doctor, Deeb's parents want him to change his lifestyle habits in order to please himself. He hurts himself more than anybody else by ignoring his diabetes, and his parents ache for him to realise that.

"He has to find his own motivation. Something within him has to give him the necessary willpower. But in the meantime, as much as he wishes we'd leave him alone, we can't! We're too afraid he will gain weight again, or just ignore this entire situation," says Aida.

The strength Deeb seeks has proven hard to come by. Aida understands some of the difficulties. As a child, Deeb wasn't always overweight; he was a tiny, skinny baby up until he was five years old or so. And his mother was always urging him to eat.

"I blame myself, I do. We shouldn't have made his weight such an issue. When he began gaining weight, we all made such a big fuss of our beautiful, healthy, chubby baby boy. It was only when he was in third or fourth grade, when I couldn't find clothes his size, that I realised he was much bigger than other children his age."

Kameel, preferring to speak of Deeb's diabetes rather than his own, feels that he and Aida have tried everything they can with Deeb. They have sent Deeb to dieticians, personal trainers, a psychologist and even an acupuncturist. Deeb was only in the sixth grade when he had his first dietician and first gym membership. Nevertheless, the young man's parents will continue trying.

"We want him to take responsibility for his actions," says Kameel. He shakes his head, and takes another drag of his cigarette, and continues explaining the dilemma he and his wife face with their son. Kameel tries to instil two important values in his son: health and education. At this point, however, Deeb's studies have lost their importance in relation to Deeb's health. "What's the point of him excelling in his studies if his health is deteriorating," says Kameel. Deeb uses the excuse that he has to study and concentrate on schoolwork instead of taking the time to exercise, and that is not acceptable to Kameel. Deeb's parents are adamant that Deeb will have to adopt a healthy lifestyle of exercise and good food choices to regulate his blood sugar levels and control his diabetes himself.

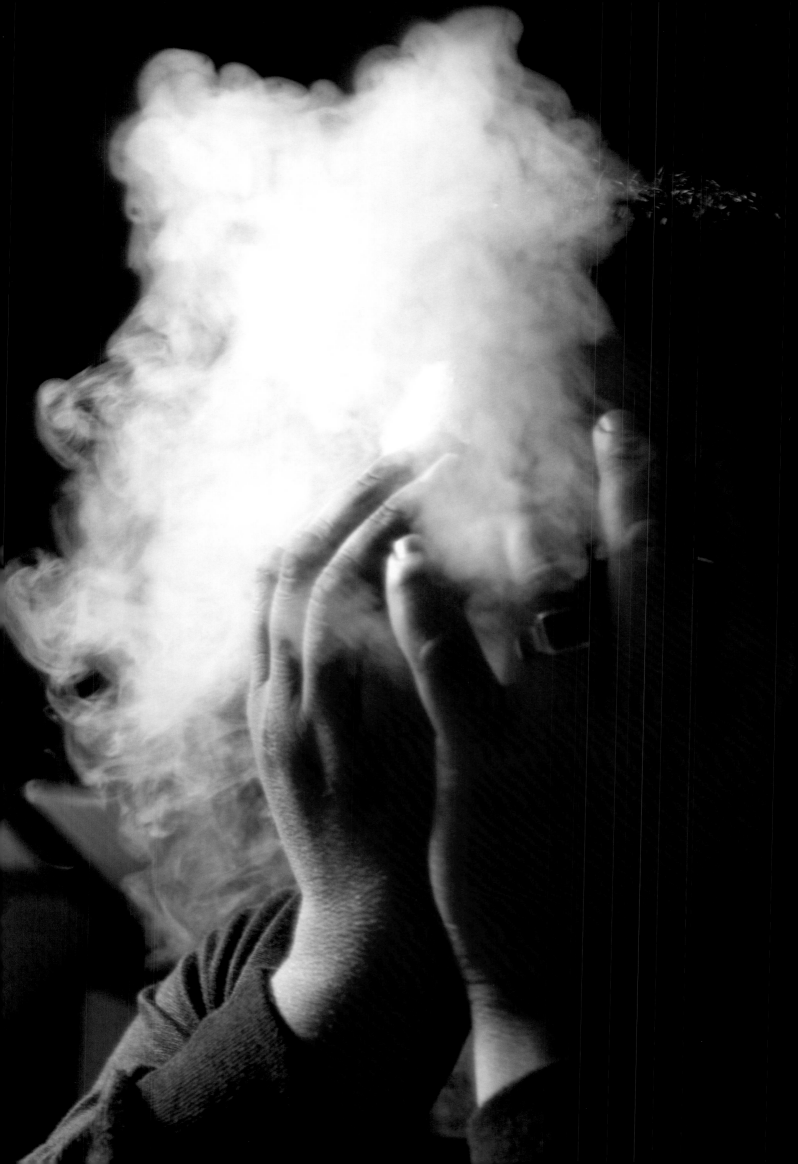

Deeb's father has type 2 diabetes himself. He is a chain smoker and although he claims an indifference towards sweets and sugar and describes himself as a sensible eater, his wife has her own thoughts on the matter.

"They're both driving me crazy, Kameel and Deebo," says Aida, throwing her hands up in the air in frustrated anger. "Kameel thinks he's doing well, but he's just tricking us and tricking himself. He'll eat healthy for two or three days, then he'll join heads with Deeb and cook something outrageously greasy and heavy. He thinks just because he uses Equal[2] in his tea instead of sugar, then he's on the right track."

Kameel definitely disagrees, explaining that he has lost 10 or 11 kilos over the past seven months, a feat he has accomplished gradually and almost subconsciously. "I was feeling fatigued from the little bit of weight I had put on," explained Kameel, a cigarette in one hand and a string of rosary beads in the other. "I really feel normal right now, I feel I have no problem with my diabetes. I have normal blood pressure and no health complaints! I know I should exercise, but I don't." He pauses to allow the coughing fit that has taken a hold of him to pass by. He then looks up, a resigned smile on his face. "And I've been smoking for too long to quit now; I just can't."

Deeb sighs and cracks his knuckles again, a habit he is prone to when he is nervous. "All I can do, really, is just pray for myself and for my father. Every difficulty in a person's life is there for a reason; God has a plan for us all."

SPIRITUAL BELONGING

The priest's forceful words resonate from the loudspeakers mounted throughout the church, and Deeb hangs on his every word. Every now and then he gives a tiny nod, agreeing with what he hears.

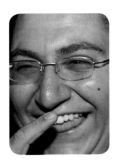

Today, Deeb's life is as full as ever. A typical day includes driving lessons early in the morning, classes that last until mid-afternoon, and from now on, he promises, vigorous exercise in the afternoon, before settling down for some studying followed by time with his friends in the evenings.

And, of course, there's church. On Saturday nights, Deeb attends the service at the new Sacred Heart of Jesus Church built in 2000. That Saturday, dressed in jeans and a navy T-shirt, he spends some time greeting his friends and joking with them outside the church before they all file in.

Deeb's blue trainers make no sound as he finds a place in one of the pews. He crosses himself before the altar, and then settles down, pushing his glasses back up onto his nose and flipping his hymnbook open to the right page.

The familiar look of peaceful serenity is back in his blue-green eyes, as he listens carefully to the priest's sermon. Ironically, the health of individuals is mentioned by the priest, who is telling his congregation that every person has an obstacle or difficulty he or she must overcome, whether in life, in health, in education, in work or in any other context. One must never give up. The strength to overcome the most difficult of hardships can always be found, within and around us.

While he listens to the sermon, Deeb's eyes glisten with barely repressed emotion. The priest's forceful words resonate from the loudspeakers mounted throughout the church, and Deeb hangs on his every word. Every now and then he gives a tiny nod, agreeing with what he hears. And as the sermon ends and the music of the next hymn fills the church, Deeb's eyelids lower, slowly, and he joins in the singing.

One cannot help but sense in Deeb a deep desire for acceptance and a search for a sense of belonging. Although he is always either joking about his weight or laughing heartily when someone teases him about it, he does so because he wants people to find him fun and likeable. When taken in a serious context, Deeb used to hate talking about his obesity or his diabetes, and avoided the subject at all costs. Now, however, Deeb seems to have grasped the importance of dealing with his health problems. He understands the danger posed by diabetes if it is ignored and neglected. He would rather have diabetes as a friend than as an enemy.

[1] Mechatronics is a type of engineering that deals with control systems and robotics; a specialisation in machines that use robotic systems.

[2] Equal is an alternative to sugar. Each serving of Equal has zero calories and less than one gram of carbohydrates.

Happy

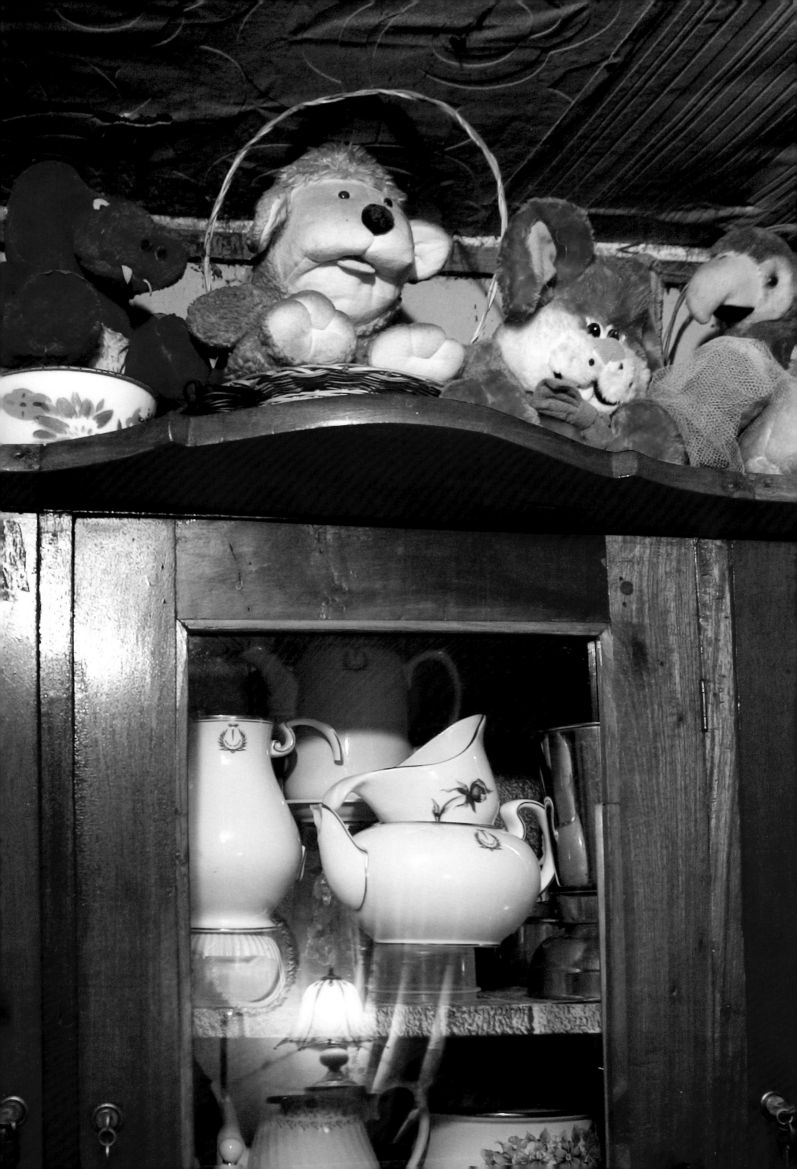

Happy George Matanje

Holding back the tears is a bit hard in Tanzania. Happy is one of many children with diabetes whose parents cannot afford to buy insulin on a regular basis, let alone glucometers and strips. They are forced to trek to hospitals and clinics in order to test blood sugar levels. After eating, the quiet, inactive and withdrawn girl that was Happy miraculously becomes a vivacious, chattering and lively child. Happy's parents cannot afford wholesome meals or regular snacks for their growing daughter. Controlling her diabetes is so hard for them. And yet, they will never give up.

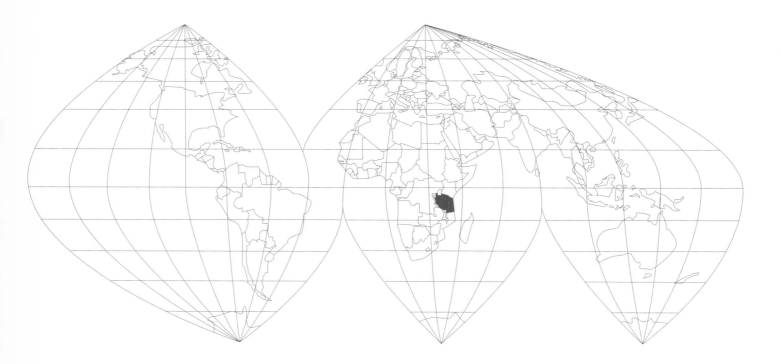

TANZANIA

Tanzania shares its border with Kenya, Uganda, Rwanda, Burundi, the Congo, Zambia, Malawi and Mozambique. Its climate varies from tropical along the coast to temperate in the highlands.

Despite its natural resources of hydropower, tin, phosphates, iron ore, coal, diamonds, gemstones, gold, natural gas and nickel, the country is poor and prone to severe flooding on the central plateau during the rainy seasons. Tanzania's main exports are gold, coffee, cashew nuts, manufactures and cotton.[1]

STATUS Republic
POPULATION 36,766,356 [2]
PEOPLE WITH DIABETES 379,000 [3]
LANGUAGES Swahili, Kiunguju, English, Arabic
RELIGIONS Christian, Muslim, Bahai, indigenous beliefs

[1] The country information is summarized from The Times Atlas of the World - Consice Edition, 1996.

[2] U.S. Census Bureau, International Data Base, September 30, 2004.

[3] International Diabetes Federation, 2004.

"I know I am sick with something; it's called diabetes."

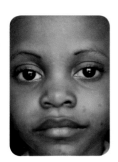

The whirring fan in the corner is doing little to alleviate the oppressive heat. Most of the twenty or so diabetes patients in the small room have taken off their tattered slippers to press the hot soles of their feet to the cool cement floor of the clinic. Outside, the rain is pouring down, adding to the intense humidity.

Inside they are waiting, patients of all ages. A baby suckling in his mother's arms, a forlorn grandmother with her weary hands clasped before her, a curious toddler huddled close to his thin mother, a couple of teenage girls sitting very still in the corner, a young father holding his small girl in his arms; all of them waiting, their eyes on one person.

Sister Elizabeth Licoco, in her crisp nurse's uniform, is first dealing with an older woman who has just walked in with a question about her diabetes. The old woman has recently been diagnosed and Sister Elizabeth is trying to comfort her, with her kind eyes and patient smile.

Eventually, the Sister turns to her waiting patients. Some have trekked all the way to the Muhimbili Diabetes Clinic only to have their blood sugar levels tested, since none have their own glucometers. Others have come to listen to one of Sister Elizabeth's educational talks, many of which are about living with diabetes. Still others have come to watch a demonstration on how to use an insulin pen. Although none of them actually *have* a pen, they *might* get one some day, and there is no harm in being prepared. And certainly some, unable to afford the needed dose of the day, have come asking for insulin.

One by one, their stories unravel. A young woman has taken her 10-year-old girl out of school, unable to afford both the insulin *and* the expensive school uniform.

A desperate mother tells how her 12-year-old daughter has been constantly in and out of hospital because of extremely high blood sugar levels. The girl has been skipping her insulin injections for the simple reason that the family is unable to afford her insulin.

The mother of a 14-year-old boy refuses to allow her son to play in the street with his friends, afraid he might cut or injure himself. If a cut is infected or does not heal properly, he will have to go to hospital. Keeping him from playing at all, she explains, makes life so much easier.

Finally, there is the story of the young father and his tiny, five-year-old girl. George has not yet sent his daughter, Happy, to nursery school. She is too young to know what is best for her, and he is concerned that she will gorge herself on the sweets, candies and ice creams that all the other children will be eating. She won't know when to say no, and her teacher might not look out for her.

"I worry that when I send Happy to school, her teacher may not take care of her the way I do," says George.

AFFORDING DIABETES

II am scared. What will happen if one day I cannot give my daughter her insulin?"

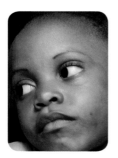 Five-year-old Happy George Matanje has had type 1 diabetes for two years. She lives with her parents and four-month-old brother, Boniface, in Dar es Salaam, Tanzania's impoverished capital. Happy's mother, Tunzo, works as a sales clerk at an auction market from seven in the morning until seven in the evening, every day of the week except Sunday. The little girl spends most of her time with her firefighter father, George, who works in shifts at the firehouse and sees more of his children than his wife.

"Tunzo and I noticed that Happy was losing weight and we took her to the hospital. She was always drinking water and had to urinate a lot. We knew something was wrong with her," says George. His daughter usually naps for two hours every afternoon, but George noticed it was getting increasingly difficult to wake Happy up from her sleep. The young parents had no choice but to bundle their daughter up and take her to a nearby private hospital.

There, after a doctor in the emergency ward had looked at Happy and given her a blood glucose test, George and Tunzo were told that she might have diabetes and that it would be better to take her to the Muhimbili Diabetes Clinic where the diagnosis could be confirmed.

Happy was immediately put on insulin and admitted into the hospital where she stayed for nine days, waiting for her condition to stabilise. Her mother stayed with her whenever she could, and her father was at the hospital as often as his shifts allowed. As George remembers it, "I stayed with Happy all day until Tunzo finished work. Then I went to work and Tunzo stayed with Happy all night. It was a difficult time."

During Happy's stay at the hospital, Tunzo and George began learning about type 1 diabetes, including insulin injections and the importance of using clean syringes. They also learned that physical exercise is crucial, just as they became acquainted with the symptoms of hypoglycaemia (low blood sugar) and hyperglycaemia (high blood sugar).

"We had no knowledge of diabetes. My mother has diabetes, but I did not know that children could have it too," says George, who had always thought diabetes was a disease affecting rich people who could afford to have sugar on a regular basis.

Tunzo remembers feeling a sense of dread while sitting with her daughter in the hospital. "We were so afraid and shocked. All the time we were thinking: How are we going to afford the medicine?"

George nods in agreement. "We are no longer scared about the diabetes as such. We learn about it and know how to take care of Happy. Diabetes is something you get used to. Our fear, now, is that we may become unable to take care of Happy some day because we cannot *afford* the insulin. That scares me. What will happen if one day I cannot give my daughter her insulin? It is so hard for us even now."

They fear that some complication of diabetes might set in, and they are especially worried about Happy's eyes. The last thing they want is for their daughter to become blind. They know that not being able to afford insulin can result in an outcome too horrible to imagine.

HAPPY'S HAVEN

IIMy favourite day is Sunday. That is the day when I can play."

Happy, with her miniature braids and big, curious eyes, gives a first impression of being a quiet and reserved little girl. She is practically invisible, sitting in the corner and staring at the television, mesmerised by the music and dancing that she loves. Her movements are slow and careful; she cannot run around the room, or through the house for that matter, for the simple reason that there is no space.

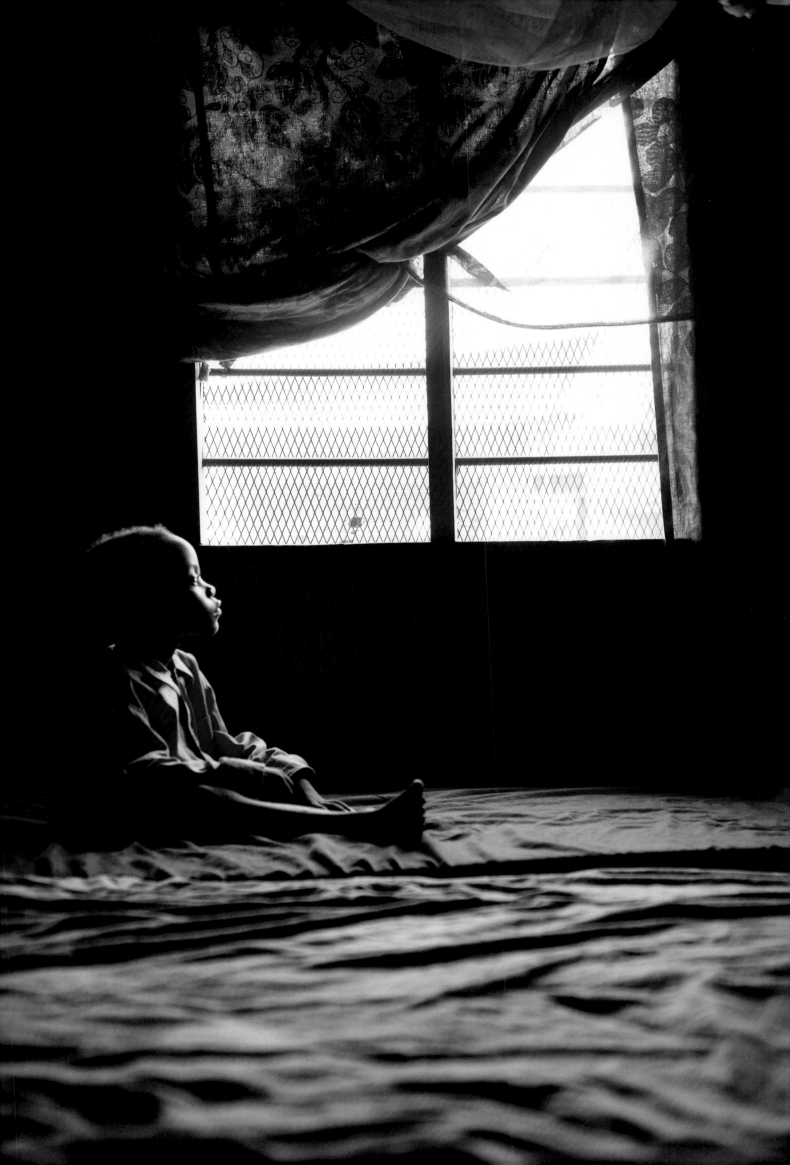

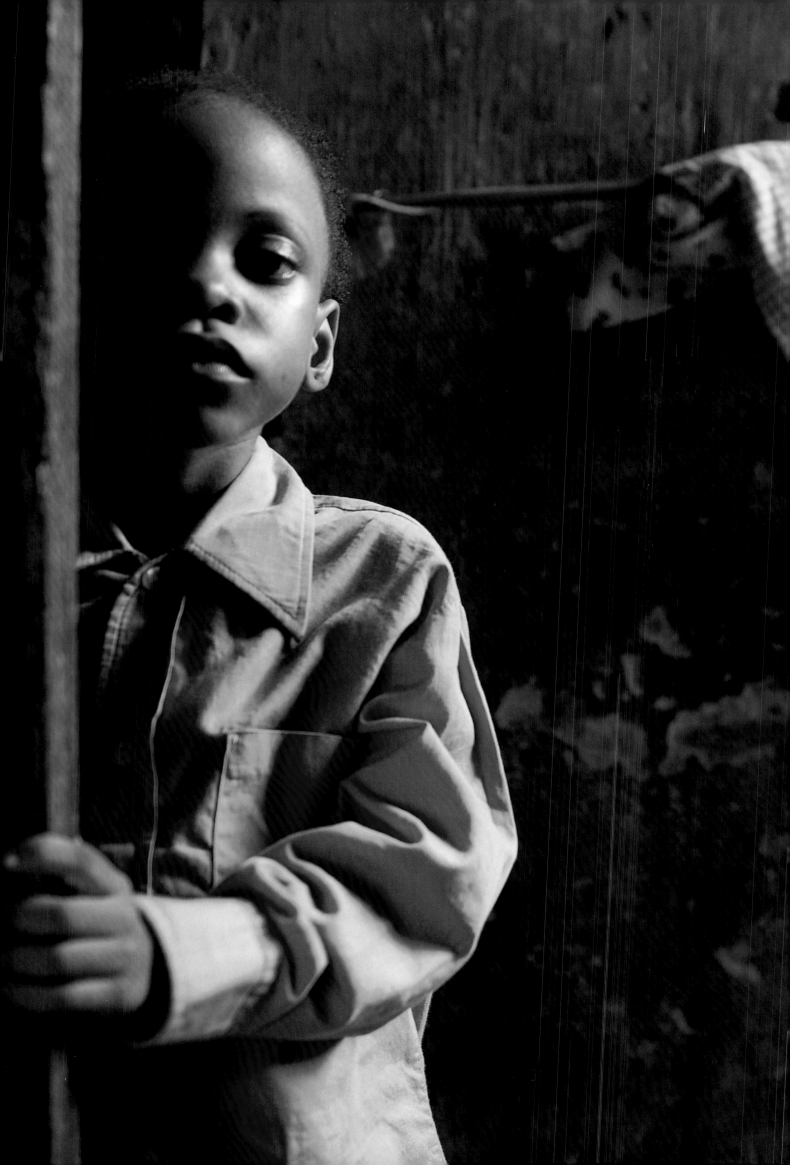

Happy's home is a testament to the poverty of Tanzania. A narrow dirt corridor filled with potholes and puddles of mud leads to two dark, confined rooms. The living-cum-dining room is decorated with wallpaper depicting snow-capped mountains and trickling streams in green forests, while the bedroom where Happy sleeps with her parents and baby brother is veiled under mosquito netting. There is no kitchen save a small fridge in the corner of the living room, empty inside but for a few tomatoes and a vial of insulin. There is very limited space to move between the cumbersome furniture and arrangements of fake flowers, and Happy has to play in the constricted hallway, crouched on the uneven ground.

The little girl gets no exercise whatsoever in the tiny apartment. She has a jump rope, but no place to use it. Playing outside in the dirt road in front of the Matanje home is not an option; it is too dangerous for a girl as young as Happy.

"I play with my toys," says Happy, in a barely audible voice, pointing at a few ragged, stuffed animals perched high on top of a cupboard. She lists the few activities she engages in during her long days. "I cook with Rosie. It's fun," she goes on, mentioning Rosie the house-girl, who takes care of Happy when her parents are at work. "And I watch television; I like the music most."

Happy thinks to herself for a few minutes. Suddenly, her eyes light up and her full lips part to reveal a shy smile. "My favourite day is Sunday. That is the day when I can play."

On Sundays, George takes his small family to his sister's home near the beach. There, Happy can roam free on the big property, playing with her eleven cousins, who all shower her with attention and care. The little girl is truly happy on Sundays, and it is amazing to witness the change in her when she is at her aunt's house.

The home is much larger than her own family's apartment and the rooms are airy and full of light. Outside is a large open area that belongs to the property, so Happy can play inside or outside – whichever her heart desires. Goats, cocks and hens roam freely in the garden, which is presided over by a large, lazy dog. A calming view of the Indian Ocean lies before the house and the beach

is just a short walk away. Happy loves to go with her cousins to watch them swim while she splashes in the water and plays in the sand. The little girl lives for her Sundays.

"Happy is trapped in the dark apartment all week. She never goes out," admits George, who feels helpless about the situation. "So we always try to go on Sunday to my sister's house, so that Happy can have some fresh air."

"We know that we must not give Happy any sugar or sweets or anything like that, because she has diabetes," says Leonard, Happy's eldest cousin. "The whole family knows it. But she is not here for sugar! She is here to play, have fun and be free in the house, and that is what we let her do."

Happy always cries when it is time to return home on Sunday afternoon. She clings to her aunt's husband, who tries to soothe the little girl and remind her that she will return again next week. He tries to distract her with a little bit of good-humoured teasing. "Now, Happy, I bought you so many soft drinks, didn't I! Which one did you choose to drink?"

Between sniffles, Happy looks up at her uncle and quietly says, "I only took one soft drink; the one that doesn't have sugar."

Her uncle laughs a deep, hearty chuckle. He lifts Happy up into the air, cradles her in his arms and looks down at her with tenderness. "It is very sad and disturbing that this small child has such a disease," he says, speaking to himself. "But still, we are very thankful to God for everything."

THE GLUCOMETER – A DESPERATE NEED

❙❙She is always either high or low, which is not good."

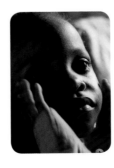

The Muhimbili Diabetes Clinic has over 3,000 diabetes patients on file, of whom only a minute proportion have a glucometer of their own. Average monthly salaries range between 50 and 60 US dollars in Tanzania, which makes it

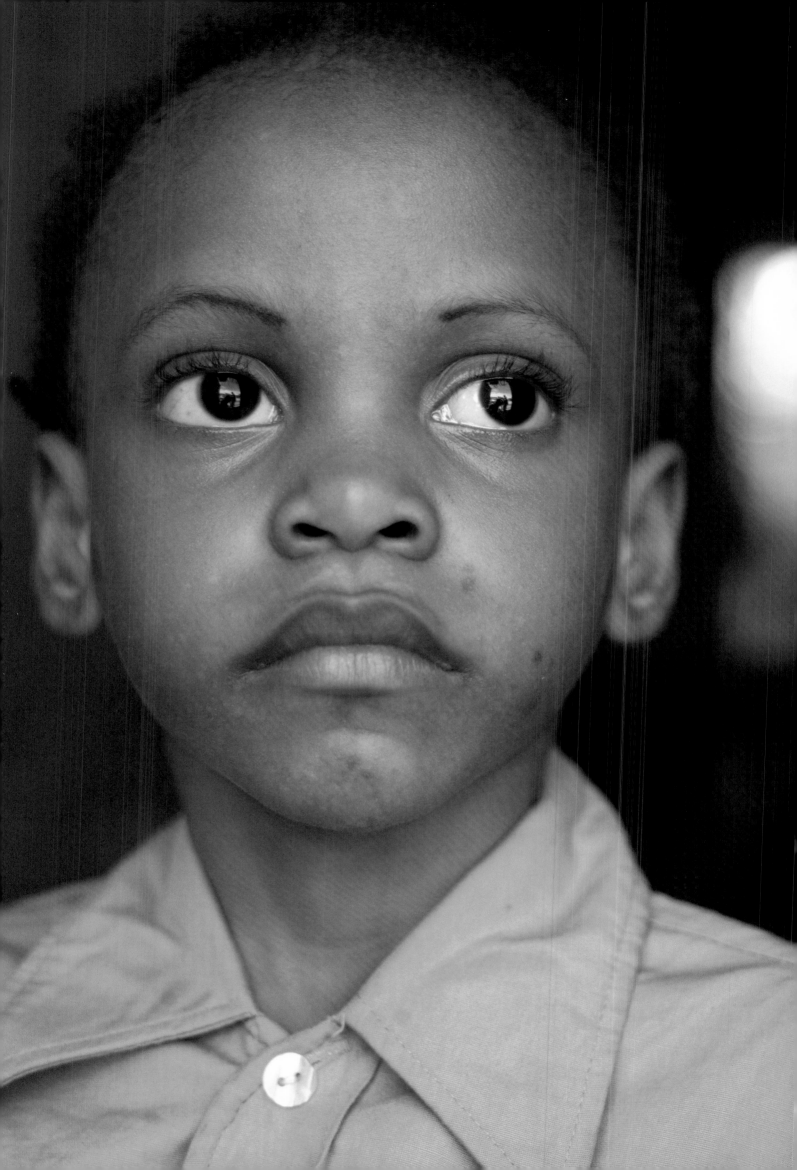

impossible to afford a glucometer, no matter whether it costs 40 dollars or 70 dollars. In addition, that price does not include the strips that must be bought regularly and quickly become another item to live without for a family facing financial hardship.

"The diabetes patients have to come to the clinic to test their blood sugar levels," says Sister Elizabeth. "When they feel that a child is not doing well, they come to the clinic and pay 1000 Tanzanian shillings, which is approximately one dollar, to test the blood glucose. This is also the case for Happy."

"It is difficult for us to pay not only for Happy's insulin but also for the testing of Happy's blood sugar," says George. "We are constantly going to hospital, which makes things very hard for us. But we need to know how Happy's blood sugar is doing to be sure that we manage her diabetes properly."

Tunzo has noticed that her daughter has recently begun to lose weight. Happy's blood sugar levels seem to be fluctuating frequently; she is either very high, always going to the bathroom and asking for a drink, or quite low, making her hungry and on edge.

"If only George and Tunzo had a glucometer, things would be so much easier for them and for Happy," says Sister Elizabeth, sighing in frustration.

"Happy needs to be monitored regularly and frequently, so we can calculate the correct dosage of insulin she needs. Proper monitoring of blood glucose levels is necessary to know if the dose is correct, if the medication is right and if the child has any problems. If Happy had a glucometer and her parents could record her readings on a chart, we would be able to explain highs and lows of blood sugar levels, and we would be able to *help* Happy. As things stand now, it is very difficult for us."

George and Happy make at least three or four trips a week to a private hospital near their home. It is more expensive to test Happy's blood sugar at the private hospital - 2000 shillings against only 1000 shillings at the Muhimbili Diabetes Clinic - but the proximity of the private hospital eliminates the need to pay the bus fare to Muhimbili.

George and Tunzo have taught the house-girl Rosie, Happy's minder, to look out for signs indicating that Happy's blood sugar is high or low. "When she is high, Happy is weak, drowsy, tired and very quiet," says George. "She is usually a talkative and active girl, so it is easy to tell when something is not right. And if she is angry and strange, then suddenly becomes sleepy, we know her blood sugar is low." Fortunately, Happy is becoming increasingly good at understanding her diabetes and usually lets her parents or Rosie know when she is high. She goes to them and explains that she is not feeling well. When she is low, however, she becomes uncharacteristically quiet, not saying a word.

If Rosie notices that Happy is falling asleep when she should not be, Rosie quickly gives Happy a little bit of glucose powder to raise her blood sugar level. Within five minutes or so, Happy seems a bit more alert, and Rosie rushes over to the neighbours next door, where she can use the phone to call either Tunzo or George.

"This has happened twice," says George. "Rosie called to tell me that Happy needed to go to the hospital and I left work and hurried home. The people at work understand that it is a matter of urgency and let me take time off when I need to. Tunzo's boss also understands, but if she leaves, she will not receive any pay for the time she is away, and we need the extra income. Tunzo returned to work only a month ago after her maternity leave following the birth of Boniface, and we were really struggling in the three months when she was not working."

Two or three times, Happy has had an emergency during the night. Once the little girl had a hypoglycaemic event while she was sleeping, and her parents were unable to wake her. It has now become a habit for George or Tunzo to get up during the night to check on Happy. If she does not stir when they shake her, her parents jump into action, hurrying to get their daughter to swallow some glucose powder in her sleep. They then carry Happy to the nearest hospital to make sure everything is all right.

"The problem is that we have no glucometer to guide us. She is always either high or low, which is not good. We have to regulate her blood sugar!" George feels almost helpless. He *knows* what must be done to control

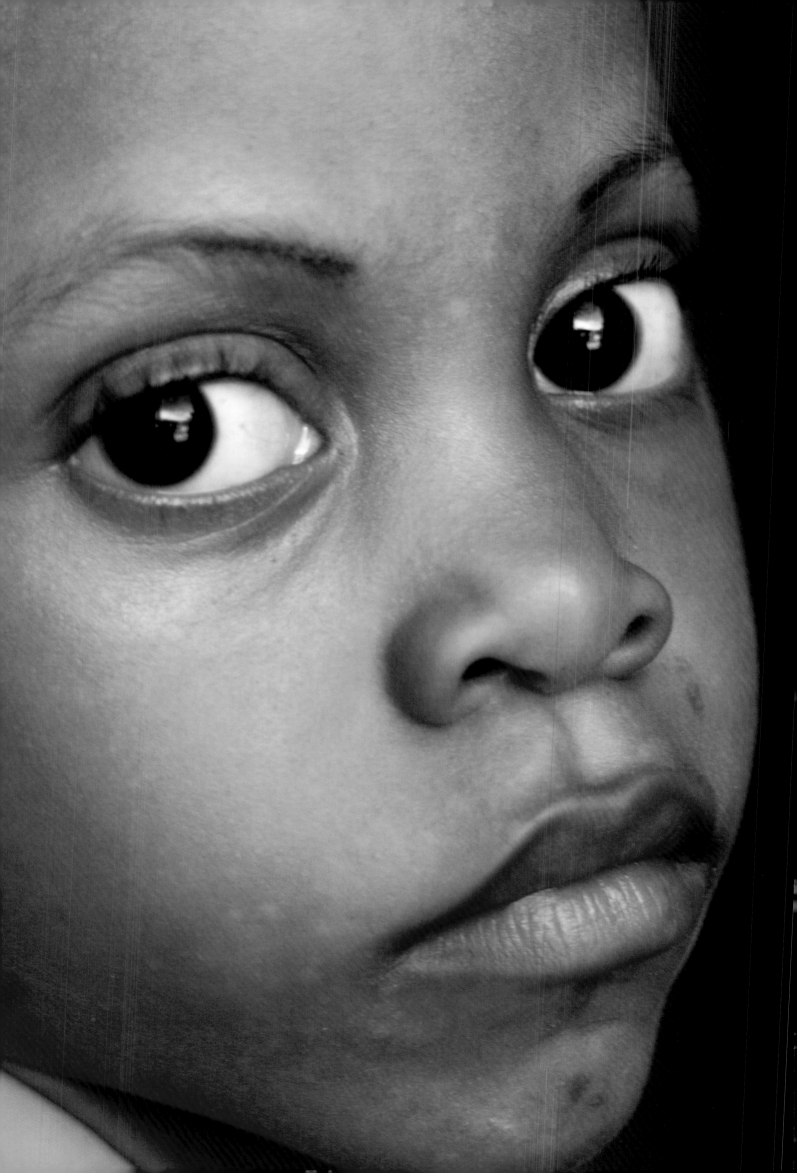

and manage his daughter's diabetes, but he does not have the means to afford it. "All we can do now is to go to a doctor and explain that Happy is not as well regulated as she should be, so that the doctor can change the dosage of insulin or try something new." On top of this, Happy does not have a regular doctor, which makes things even worse. Her parents always end up in the emergency ward, waiting for the doctor on duty to see them, whoever he or she might be. In Tanzania, the concept of a regular family physician is almost non-existent.

DREAMING OF SCHOOL

❚❚Yes, Happy, you are right. You will go to school when you are cured."

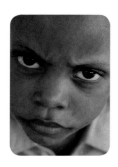

"I want to go to school! I want to be educated!" Any mention of school injects a spurt of enthusiasm in the otherwise very quiet Happy, her attention diverted from the television set and onto the subject of school. She huddles closer to Sister Elizabeth and looks up at her with adoration lighting up her eyes. "I want to be a big sister when I grow up, because the nurses have nice dresses, like Sister Elizabeth. I like their clothes."

Sending their daughter to nursery school will place an additional financial burden on the already strained George and Tunzo. "I want to send Happy to the best school, so she is well prepared for her primary education at the community schools when she turns seven," explains George. "If I send her to the best private school, she will not only get the best education but will also be treated normally, even though she has diabetes. There will be good teachers, who will look out for her and not let her be isolated or mistreated by other children because of her diabetes."

Unfortunately, the school George has in mind will cost 45,000 shillings a month, which is an impossible expense considering George's monthly salary of 70,000 shillings. "We cannot afford it, I know. But maybe I can ask for a loan from my employer. Or maybe I can borrow some money from relatives. I don't know." George falls silent.

If Happy's parents are unable to send her to this specific private school, they prefer to let her stay at home until it is time for her to go to the ordinary school rather than enrol her in a cheaper school.

"The reason is that we have already talked to the teachers at this specific school and explained to them that Happy has type 1 diabetes. The teachers are understanding and responsible. They know how to take care of Happy," says Tunzo. "In any other school, Happy's diabetes would be ignored. She cannot take care of herself. She might eat things she shouldn't. Then what will we do?"

The family's financial difficulties are making life with diabetes harder than it needs to be. A vial of insulin, which lasts for three weeks, costs 7,500 shillings. Renting the apartment costs 30,000 shillings a month, and Rosie's salary is 10,000 a month. Tunzo's job is not permanent and her salary, not always consistent, is never more than 40,000 shillings a month.

Tunzo knows her husband is doing the best he can. Many a time, Happy has said to her mother, "One day, I am going to be cured, right? And when that happens, you will let me go to school, right? Because right now, you are not letting me go to school because I am sick, right?"

All Tunzo can do is nod in agreement despite her knowledge that diabetes is a chronic illness with no cure, and say, "Yes, Happy, you are right. You will go to school when you are cured."

A HUNGRY LITTLE GIRL

❚❚I wish I could get a better house so Happy could have better ventilation and more space to play in. I wish I could make sure she had a proper diet. But sometimes towards the end of the month there is barely any food to eat."

"I like to eat! I like to eat! I am such a good eater!" The change that occurs in Happy after she has had just a little bit to eat is almost impossible to believe.

Shortly after arriving at her aunt's house on a Sunday, the quiet Happy sits down with her cousins to have a

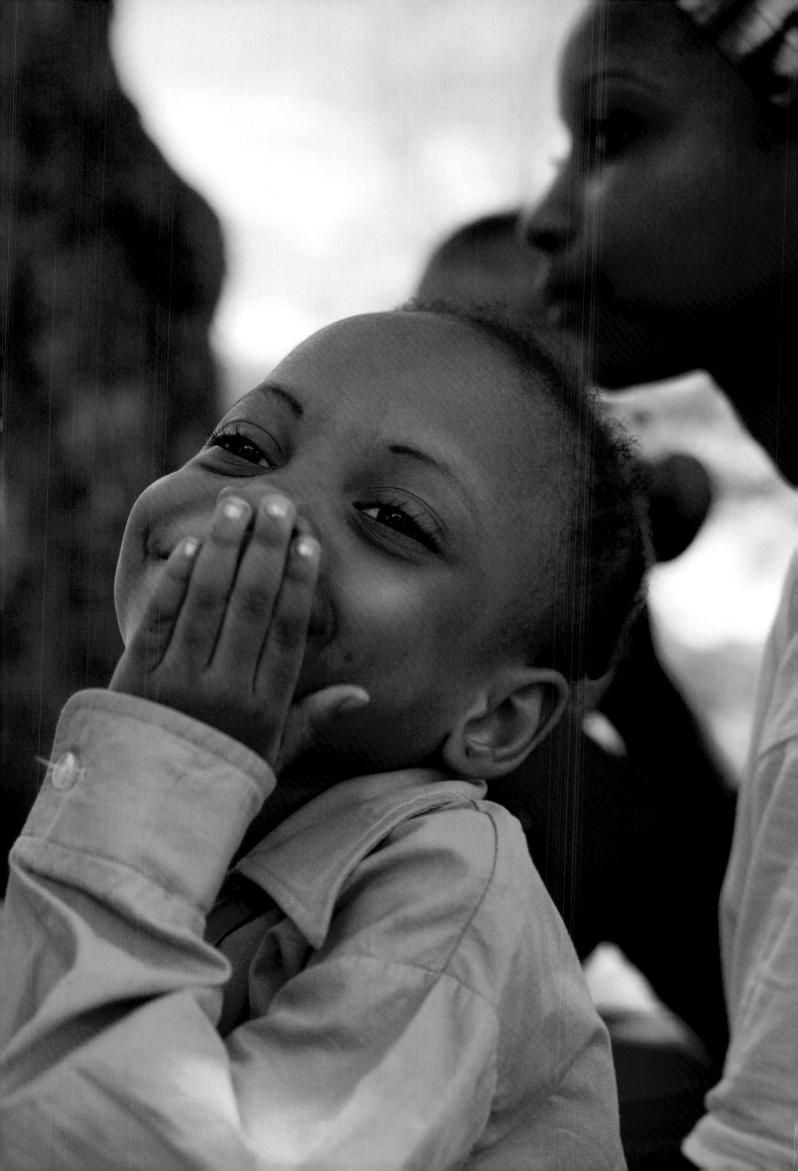

hearty lunch of rice, fresh tomatoes and plenty of chicken. Her tiny hands grasp the spoon, shovelling the food into her mouth with barely a pause between bites. Within seconds, Happy is transformed. Suddenly, the normally quiet little girl is chattering non-stop, humming and singing to herself.

A few minutes later she starts skipping. With a piece of chicken grasped tightly in her fist, she runs around the house, chewing and singing, "This meat has been given to me by God! I love this meat! It's from God! Oh and I would just love a soda right now too, to wash down this meat! I love to eat! I am such a good eater!"

George and Tunzo haltingly admit that Happy does, in fact, eat better meals on Sundays when she visits her aunt. The salty crackers that are the only snack available to her at her parents' home are quickly forgotten. Instead, Happy slurps on sugar-free soft drinks and chews on pieces of chicken, while chasing the squawking hens.

"I love milk and bananas and rice and fish and apples and peanuts," squeals Happy, displaying the talkative nature her parents know is deep within her. "Sweets? I don't like sweets. Or maybe I do! I don't know! I never have any." But that matters little to Happy, who would much rather have solid food than sweets she is not used to eating.

"If I had a better income, maybe I could take better care of my family," says George, his voice suddenly uneven and raspy. "I wish I could get a better house so Happy could have better ventilation and more space to play in. I wish I could make sure she had a proper diet. But sometimes towards the end of the month there is barely any food to eat. Meals are smaller and Happy has less to eat. She is so thin! Sometimes I can't even afford to buy milk for her because Boniface needs it too. We are living from my employer's pocket to our mouths."

A minute later George insists that they are doing fine, and the only thing they need is a little help with the expenses. They understand diabetes and they know what they need to do for Happy. He just wishes that he could at least afford to buy suitable snacks for Happy instead of resorting to glucose powder to raise her blood sugar level.

DADDY'S LITTLE GIRL

❙❙My father takes care of me. So I will be okay."

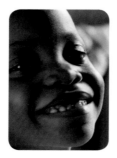

"Oh, Happy loves her daddy," says Tunzo, trying to lighten the discussion. "When Boniface was born, Happy was a little bit jealous, worried that the baby would take away her father's attention. But she knows how much her daddy loves her, and she is so sweet to her little brother, singing songs to him and dancing for him. Of course, she goes to her daddy if she needs anything. He is the one she wakes up at night if she needs some milk."

Tunzo knows that Happy has this close relationship with her father because she spends so much more time with him than with her mother. Happy barely sees her mother during the week because of Tunzo's long working hours. Tunzo would have preferred to stay at home with her daughter but has to work to bring in the second income. Nonetheless, her thoughts stay with her daughter: Whenever Happy's blood sugar level is low on a morning before Tunzo goes to work, the harried mother spends the entire day worrying about her daughter.

"Day by day, Happy is becoming more and more aware of her diabetes, but she goes to her father for understanding," says Tunzo. "She used to cry a lot whenever she had to take an insulin injection, and she also used to cry whenever her finger was pricked at the hospital so her blood sugar could be tested, but she has grown accustomed to it now and knows that we are taking care of her."

Little Happy is prone to reminding her father of her insulin shots even if she is not due for an injection anytime soon. She worries about falling sick and having to be taken to the hospital again, so she reminds her father several times a day to give her the insulin injection.

The tiny girl with expressive eyes and rare smiles sits close to her father, tickling her baby brother and leaning her head against her father's muscular arm. "I know I am sick with something; it's called diabetes," she says, looking to her father for encouragement. "It makes me sad. But my father takes care of me. So I will be okay."

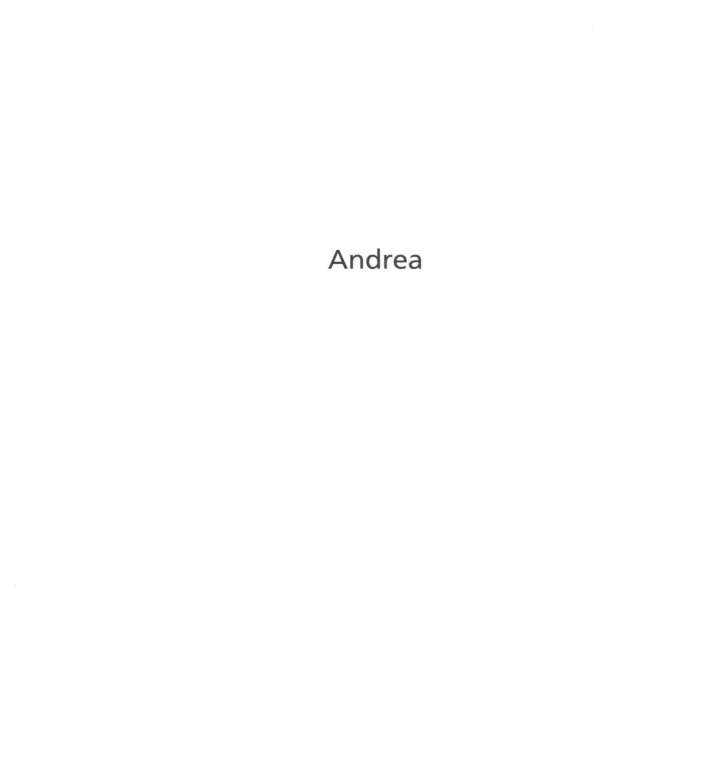

Andrea

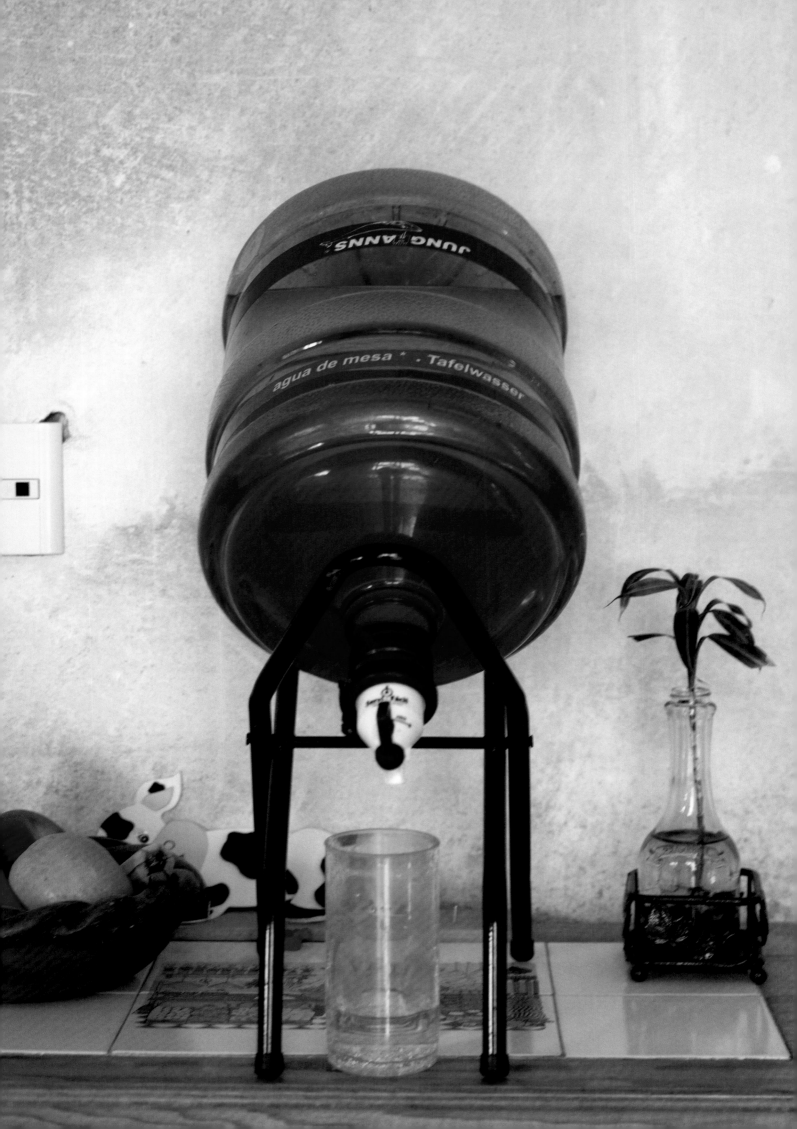

Andrea Monjarás Taméz

Andrea is a child flourishing under the firm but loving care of her parents, who have taught her since the age of four to take care of herself and her diabetes. It is amazing to see how aware this beautiful and intelligent nine-year-old is. Andrea knows that by taking care of herself, she can live her life, with all it has to offer, and she does not want to waste a minute missing out on the beauty of living.

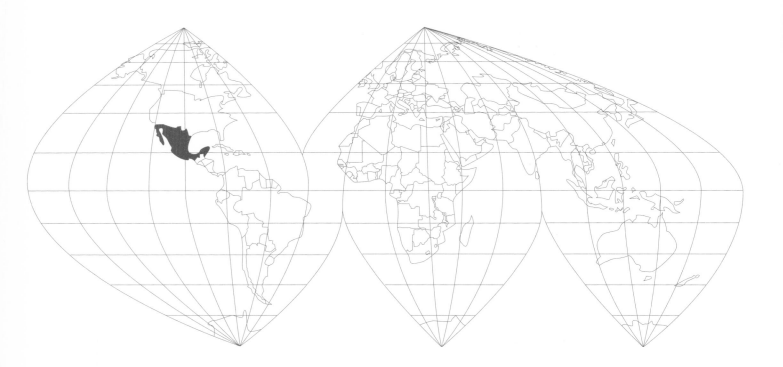

MEXICO

From its borders with Guatemala and Belize in the south, to the USA border in the north, Mexico covers a wide range of climates: hot and humid in the lowlands, warm in the centre plateaus and cool in the Sierra Madre mountain range, with a desert-like climate in the north and heavy rainfalls in the south. Mexico City is the second largest in the world, with over 22 million inhabitants.

[1] The country information is summarized from The Times Atlas of the World - Consice Edition, 1996.

A quarter of the Mexican workforce is involved in agriculture, with the main exports being coffee, fruits and vegetables. Timber production is also important for exports. Mexico is rich with minerals, such as zinc, copper, lead and sulphur. Mexico is also the leading producer of silver, as well as one of the world's leading producers of oil. [1]

[2] U.S. Census Bureau, International Data Base, September 30, 2004.

STATUS Federal Republic
POPULATION 106,202,903 [2]
PEOPLE WITH DIABETES 4,400,000 [3]

[3] International Diabetes Federation, 2004.

LANGUAGES Spanish, Mayan
RELIGIONS Roman Catholic, Protestant

"It is my thing. I have to deal with it."

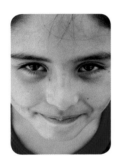

Quickly and confidently, her moves nimble and careful, she grabs a branch and hoists herself up into the lush tree. With firm grips and footholds, she uses the irregular branches like the rungs of a ladder. Soon her father has to shade his eyes to look up at her brown, grinning face peering down through the leaves. The bright sunlight is glistening off her hair, still wet from her recent dip in the swimming pool. She perches in the tree like a young monkey, not worried about how she will ever get back down again. She is not the sort to waste her time with worry, for every moment of every second is taken up with *living*.

"Andrea, be careful! You got yourself up there, so you will get yourself down," bellows her father, Carlos, who believes in giving his children guidance to make the right decisions coupled with independence to learn as they grow.

Andrea laughs and pushes aside the branches of leaves to smile at the digital camera her brother, Diego, is pointing at her. After her expedition up her grandfather's tree has been well documented, she begins her descent, her father watching closely beneath her, ready to catch her if she should fall.

But, unsurprisingly, she makes it down in one piece, laughing the entire way. With her father's steady hand supporting her, Andrea jumps onto the soft grass and takes off running, turning a few cartwheels as she goes. She gives a shout along the way and looks over her shoulder to make sure her acrobatics are observed by her family.

The entire time, whether standing on her hands or scrambling up a tree trunk, Andrea's insulin pump, protected in its leather pouch, remains firmly attached to the waistband of her shorts. It does not budge, and Andrea, who has type 1 diabetes, pays no attention to it.

AN EMERGENCY

❚❚We had been suffering for weeks, not knowing what was wrong with our daughter ... she couldn't tell us what was wrong!"

Nine-year-old Andrea Monjarás Taméz is Carlos and Ivonne's middle child; her brother Diego is almost 11, and Fernanda, Andrea's trusting devotee, is six. The family live in Cuernavaca, a town located 1,542 metres above sea level in the mountains south of Mexico City. Although Cuernavaca is only 45 minutes' drive from Mexico City, the second largest city in the world, the two are worlds apart. The colonial town, known for its 'eternal spring' climate, has long been a retreat for the capital's more affluent citizens, and because of its mild weather and green areas, Carlos and his wife also find Cuernavaca ideal for raising a family.

Despite the seemingly pastoral environment, things have not always been easy for the family. In June 1997, when Andrea was only eighteen months old, her parents noticed that something was wrong. She lost weight at an alarming speed, urinated frequently and was always thirsty, never refusing anything to drink.

"We did not know what was wrong with her," says Carlos, describing those hard days. "There was only one paediatrician in our town. We lived in the town of Cocoyoc at the time, not far from Cuernavaca. We consulted doctors all the time, but no one could tell us what was wrong with Andrea."

As the story unfolds, Ivonne's face becomes drawn, while Carlos gestures with his hands. "One night, we didn't sleep. Andrea, just a little baby, was throwing up all night long. We did not know what to *do* for her. She just kept drinking and drinking water! Ivonne was going crazy, and I was trying very hard to stay in control, but we were terrified."

Very early the next morning, Carlos and Ivonne hurried to call their local paediatrician, anxious to give Andrea some relief. When the doctor showed no concern and told them to pass by his clinic later that morning after ten o'clock, their fragile patience snapped.

"We had been suffering for weeks, not knowing what was wrong with our daughter," says Carlos, as he recalls the memories with difficulty. "She was just a baby, so she couldn't tell us what was wrong! I called a friend, who called a friend, and soon we were on our way to Mexico City, to the emergency ward, where we were promised a doctor would be waiting for us to see Andrea."

"My husband drove like a crazy man that day, and I held Andrea in my arms," says Ivonne, adding that Diego sat quietly in the backseat, aware that something was seriously wrong with his sister. "Andreas's head was flopping backwards and she was barely moving," she recalls. "We were frantic with worry."

They pulled up at the hospital's emergency entrance. A doctor was waiting, ready to take Andrea and give her parents some answers. Carlos and Ivonne waited, Diego seated between them, and shortly after the doctor came back to ask them a simple question: "Have you heard about something called diabetes?" Carlos and Ivonne, struck speechless, could do nothing but stare in shock.

NEVER HAVING KNOWN ANY OTHER WAY

//Andrea has grown up with diabetes – she has never had the chance to compare her life with anything else."

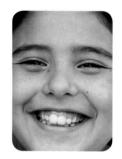

For an individual with normal blood glucose levels, anything between 70 and 110 milligrams of sugar per decilitre (mg/dl) of blood is acceptable. When Andrea was admitted into hospital that day, her blood sugar level was over 900 mg/dl, which put her in a critical condition. She could have collapsed into a coma. Recalling how close they were to that point is almost too much for her parents to bear.

"Of course I don't remember any of it! I was just a *baby*," says Andrea, laughing at the idea of such drama. "When Mama and Papi talk about it, they always look so sad and worried. But it's not a big deal! Everything is okay now, and I am always okay and fine," she exclaims, her head nodding vigorously.

Andrea is somewhat curious as to why anyone would want to talk about her diabetes. She thinks the whole discussion is rather irrelevant for the simple reason that she never dwells on it. "I know I have something called diabetes, but I've *always* had it! Since it was always there, I don't think about it much; I just do what I have to do to take care of myself."

Andrea has never known a single day when diabetes was not a part of her life. As a result, living with it comes easily and naturally.

"Andrea has grown up with diabetes – she has never had the chance to compare her life with anything else," explains her father. "Being aware of it, eating correctly,

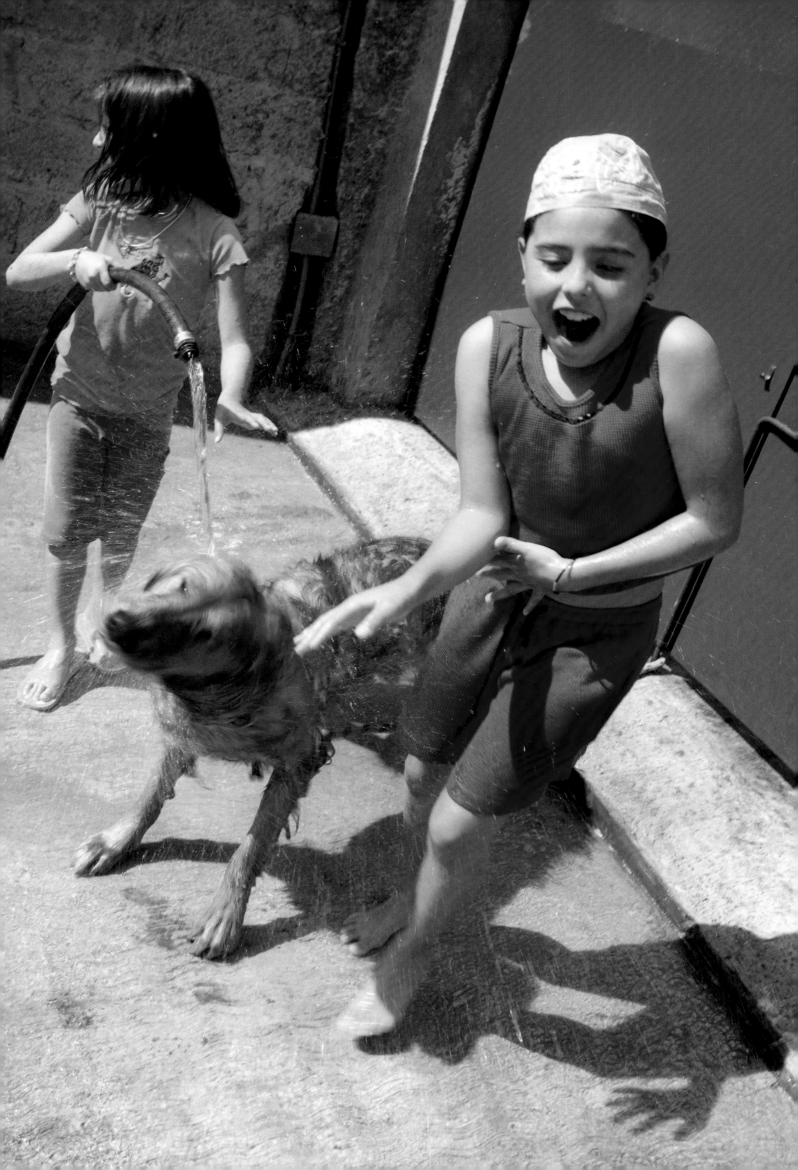

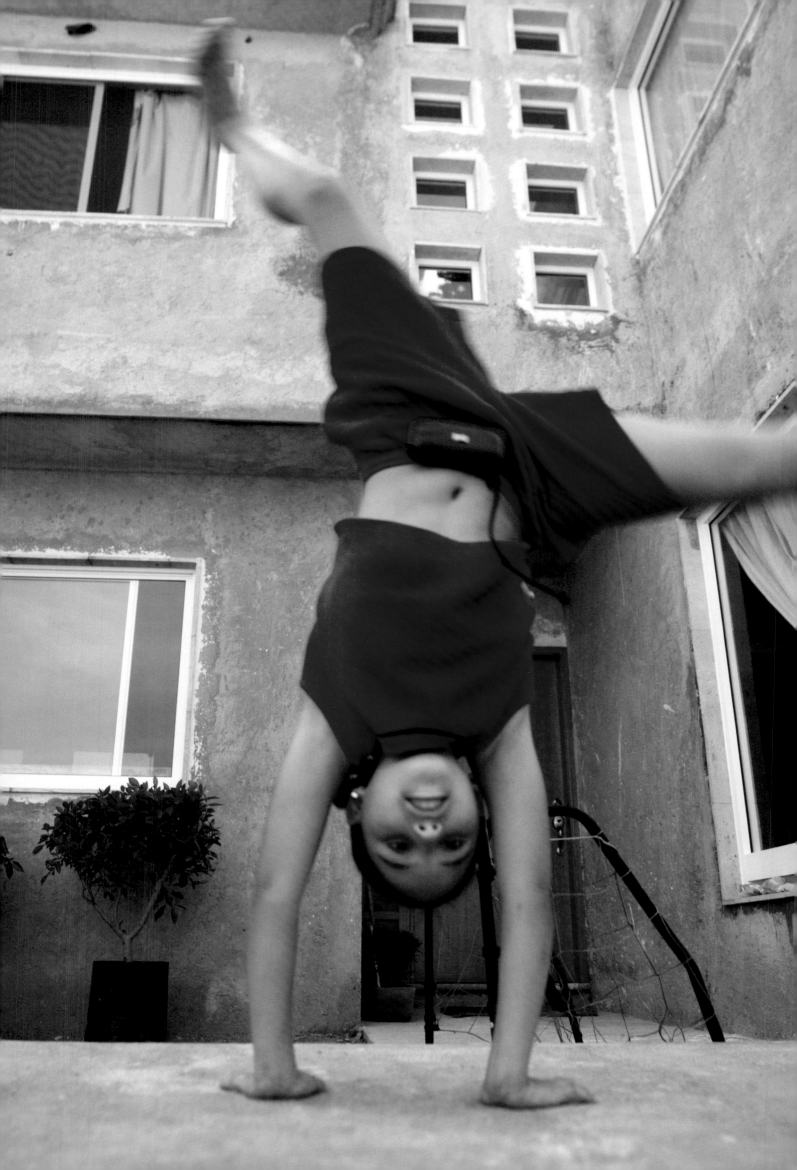

measuring her blood sugar levels at least eight times a day and taking her insulin have always been a part of her life. To her, it is normal and routine," says Carlos. "And like she says, it's no big deal."

Andrea has her own way of describing what living with diabetes means to her. "I take care of diabetes because it is part of my body and I have to take care of my body. It's just like brushing my teeth. I take care of my teeth and I take care of my diabetes."

"DEAL WITH IT"

❙❙We knew from the very beginning that this diabetes thing would *not* be allowed to take over Andrea's life."

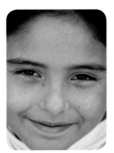

Day by day, Carlos and Ivonne learned how to take care of their baby daughter and her diabetes. At first it was difficult, confusing and terrifying, and Ivonne admits to having spent hours crying. "It was so hard, giving her the very first injection myself. I didn't want to hurt my baby, and I knew I had to do it for her own good, but it was *so hard*."

Luckily, the Monjarás family have a special outlook on life that helped them find the right way to deal with the situation. "We knew from the very beginning that we would *not* allow the diabetes to take control of Andrea's life," says Carlos firmly. Hence, Andrea has never been treated differently by her parents, nor has she ever used her condition to get what she wants or to attract attention. The three children – Diego, Andrea and Fernanda – are treated equally. Their parents would not have it any other way.

"It is my thing. I have to deal with it. If my Mama and Papi are not here to remind me, I check my blood sugar myself and I make sure my pump gives me the right amount of insulin," says Andrea. She sprints off to the kitchen to wave at a little white board resting against the wall. On it is a chart of numbers written in a green marker and attached behind a magnet is a shuffle of papers.

"This is where I look if I have questions or if I am wonder-

ing about something. I can look up what kind of food and how much of it I can eat or how much insulin I have to take depending on my blood sugar level. My parents prepared this for me, so I can take care of myself," she says triumphantly.

Carlos and Ivonne taught Andrea how to inject herself with insulin at the young age of four, long before she ever had the pump.

"We want her to be prepared for anything," explains Carlos. "We don't want the diabetes to prevent her from doing whatever she wants, so we want her to be ready. That is our way," he explains. Carlos and Ivonne's strategy has paid off. Andrea does whatever she has to do to control her diabetes and take care of herself and looks to her parents for guidance whenever she needs it.

"I have to say I am so impressed by my daughter," says Carlos, his eyes shining with pride. Andrea's strong character and love of life comfort her parents, who truly feel they need not worry about their intelligent, careful daughter. "She has never cried over her diabetes; can you believe it? I don't remember Andrea ever crying because she had to have an injection or because she had to have a check-up or could not eat two sandwiches instead of just one." Carlos pauses for a moment and then speaks as if he is thinking aloud; "Maybe it's because all this is normal to her. Maybe things are easier for her because her diabetes came when she was so young and she has grown up with it. I don't know. But whatever it is, we are very thankful."

ANDREA'S TREASURES

❙❙I guess a perfect day for me, more or less, is playing with Scrubby and giving him a wash."

"I love you, I love you, señor Scrubby; I love you!" Andrea buries her head in the gleaming fur of her golden retriever, Scrubby, and hugs him ferociously. The dog shifts uncomfortably for a moment, seemingly not able to breathe, but his tail wags hysterically.

"There is a special connection between Andrea and that dog," says Carlos, shaking his head. Apparently, Scrubby is devoted to one mistress: Andrea. She, in turn, can

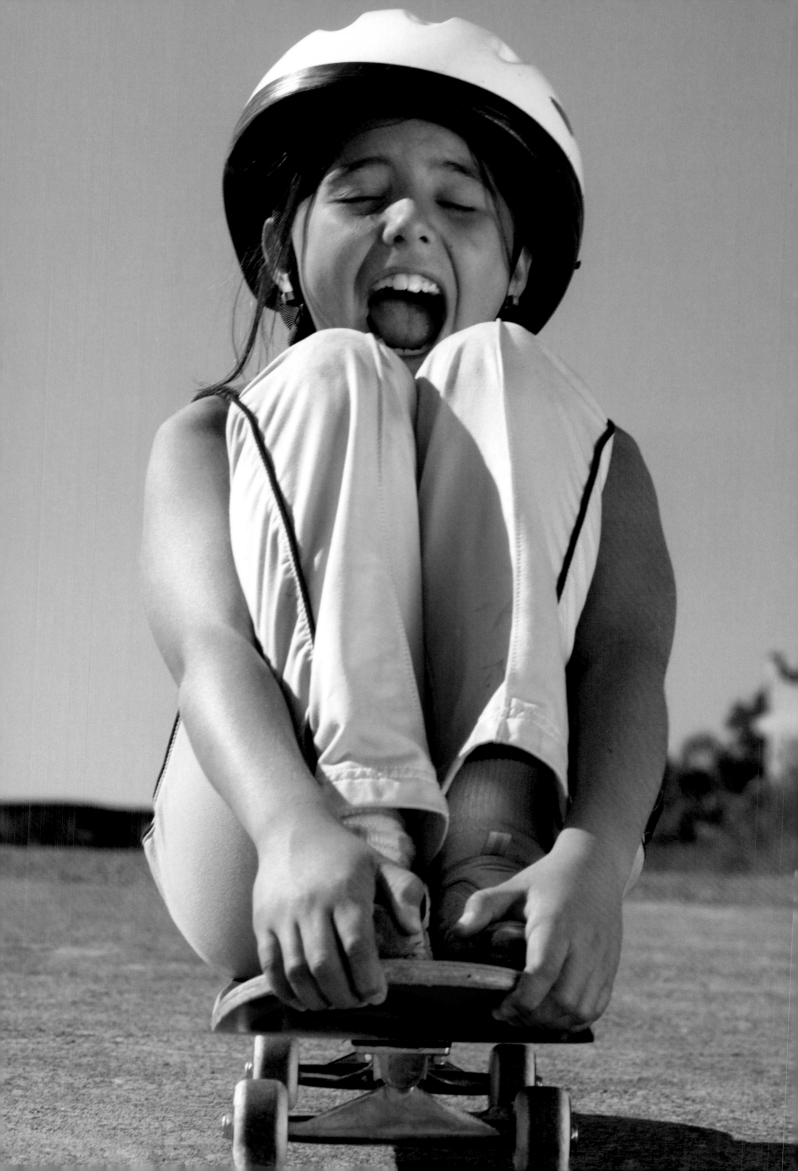

spend hours doing nothing more than just *being* with her dog. Her love of animals has fuelled a desire in her to become a veterinarian; either that, she says, or she would like to be a pilot like her father.

"I guess a perfect day for me is playing with Scrubby and giving him a wash," says Andrea, while Fernanda vigorously nods in agreement in her shadow. It is a natural sight to spot the two girls in shorts, kerchiefs in their hair, carrying bottles of dog shampoo out to the waiting Scrubby. In no time, water and soap is everywhere, accompanied by laughter and shrieks.

In quieter moments, Andrea connects with Peluchin, a small, scruffy black teddy bear with an orange hat and glitter mixed into his fur. It was the last present Andrea received from her grandmother before the old woman died. The teddy nestles in the crook of Andrea's arm, as she runs around the house playing and singing, stopping to draw a colourful picture or to brush a Barbie doll's hair. Peluchin, however, is flung aside when Andrea decides to play on her skateboard.

"Most of all, a really, really perfect day is going to Lolo's house," says Andrea, describing the family's weekend visits to Andrea's grandfather's house. There, the children splash in the pool and play. While Diego and Fernanda spend most of their time lying in the hammock, playing with their uncle and climbing trees, Andrea turns cartwheels and practises her gymnastics – a sport she has been pursuing avidly for almost a year now.

When the Monjarás family arrive at Lolo's house, there are bowls of snacks lined up neatly on a garden table. Diego and Fernanda help themselves to chips, while Andrea runs off to play. Later, when she has exhausted herself with swimming and running, she helps herself to a few chips, careful not to have too many.

"My favourite food is pizza, actually," she says, taking a sip from the small glass of sugar-free diet soda Ivonne has poured for her.

FOOD CONTROL

"I don't feel bad about having diabetes, but sometimes I feel I can't eat what I want, like candy, while my brother

and sister can eat *anything* they want," says Andrea, finally admitting to one aspect of diabetes that gets to her. Sometimes, the growing girl would like to have an extra slice of pizza or gorge herself on sweets instead of fruit. However, in such moments Andrea knows she has to make the healthy choice and does so with only a tiny grumble.

Ivonne does not make any special food for Andrea; the entire family eat the same food whenever they sit down for a meal. While Andrea's portions are small and filling, her snacks are more frequent than those of her brother and sister and mostly consist of fruit. She drinks a glass of milk with a spoonful of honey if her blood sugar levels drop slightly.

"I was a devil for Halloween this year," exclaims Andrea, "And I didn't eat all my candy like Diego and Fernanda!" Andrea came back home from trick-or-treating and hid away all her candy, allowing herself only one, small candy. Her bag of treats lasted her for weeks; she only ate a chocolate or a sweet when she knew she could. To her, eating too much candy is not healthy for anybody. Diabetes does not have *that* much to do with it.

Although Andrea is never treated differently and eats with the rest of the family, there are special occasions. When Ivonne and Carlos throw a Halloween party or for that matter any other sort of gathering, they make sure that there are some special treats for Andrea to enjoy.

"We don't want her to feel left out, so we get some sugar-free candies, and there are always some sugar-free drinks around too," says Carlos. "This means that she feels she is normal and part of what is going on."

At school, Andrea always has a nutritious snack in her lunchbox. If she feels she is becoming tired or anxious, she knows that her blood sugar levels have dropped, and she quietly and inconspicuously reaches for a drink of juice or piece of fruit.

"That little girl is a delight to have in the classroom," says Andrea's fourth-grade teacher. "She is friends with everyone and she is always laughing and smiling. Sometimes I have to tell her to quiet down, but she is such a social little girl!" Andrea's teacher points out that very few of Andrea's friends

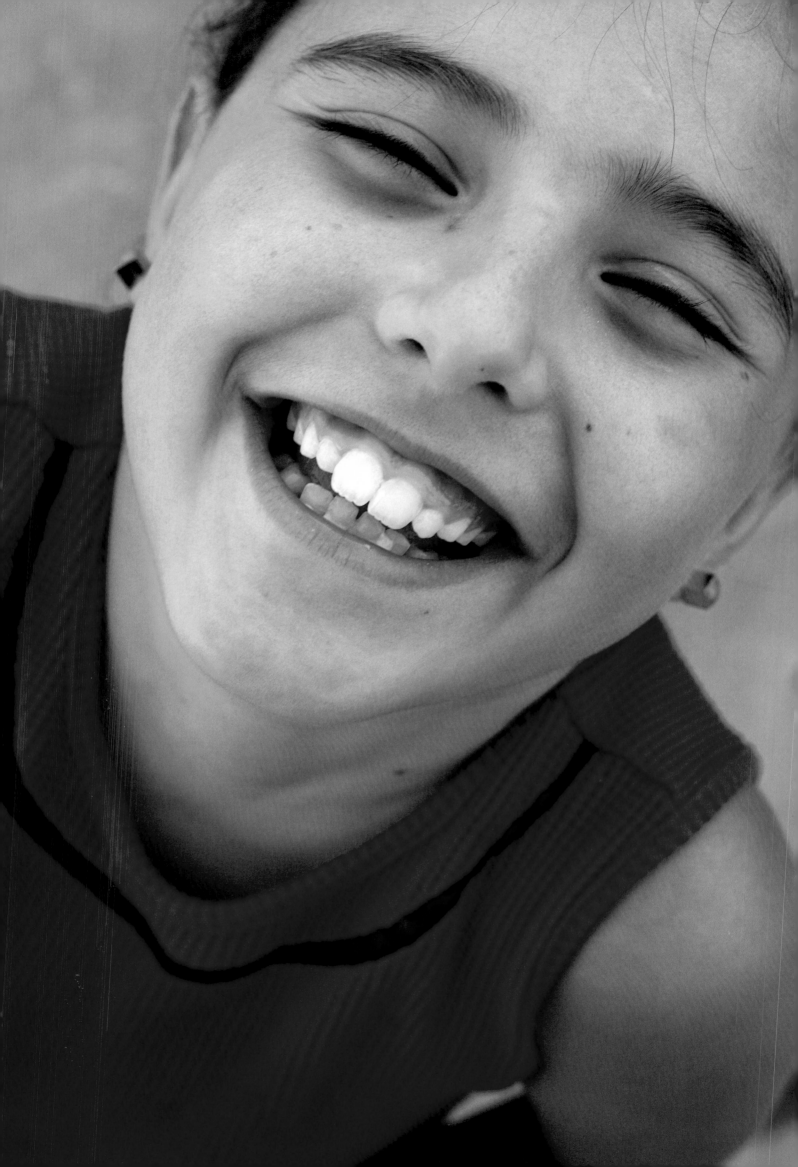

are even aware of her diabetes. She is an active participant in sports, including soccer, basketball and gymnastics. She spends her breaks like everyone else, playing and running around. Her insulin shots are non-existent now, thanks to the versatility of her pump.

"Andrea's diabetes has never been an issue at school. I never watch what she eats, because she knows herself what she should eat. She is a clever girl. I never worry about her," says her teacher.

DIFFICULTIES NONETHELESS

❚❚ Mama, I am different from everyone, right? I am different in a bad way and it's my fault, isn't it?"

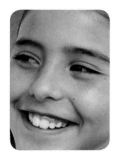

"You know, we have been very lucky with Andrea, but there have been difficult times," says Carlos. One such difficult time was just a few days after Andrea had been diagnosed and Carlos, a pilot for a Mexican airline, had to go to the United States for a month of special compulsory training. Ivonne stayed alone with her baby daughter in the hospital while Diego stayed with his grandparents. When Carlos returned, he had to rely on Ivonne to teach him everything he had to know about diabetes and about how to take care of Andrea.

These days, they regularly buy books to help them learn more and make sure they consult their doctor whenever a question arises. "All the diabetes books we read say you need to communicate well with your doctor," says Carlos. "Doctors must allow you to ask questions. We weren't getting that from our previous doctor. Although he was the best in Mexico, when it came to dealing with us as people, he was cold and reserved. And as Andrea was growing older, she was becoming more uncomfortable with him because he was a man. So we did what was best for our daughter. We found another doctor, and she is perfect for us now." It is time, they think, to find some books or leaflets on diabetes geared towards children, so Andrea can do some reading of her own.

Another difficulty encountered by Andrea's parents was

when Andrea was about five years old and began to realise she was dealing with something few others had to deal with. Andrea was in kindergarten in Cocoyoc at the time, and her teachers did not seem to take her diabetes seriously.

"We had some problems with that school. Andrea had a little emergency that had nothing to do with her diabetes, but *because* she had diabetes, the teachers panicked instead of acting responsibly and asked that Andrea be removed from the school," says Carlos, repressing the anger he feels whenever he thinks of the incident.

Ivonne and Carlos did not hesitate to leave the school, enrolling Andrea temporarily in another school in Cocoyoc while preparing to move to Cuernavaca. Andrea was frightened by the incident at school and felt that everything was her fault.

"Mama, I am different from everyone, right? I am different in a bad way and it's my fault, isn't it?" When Andrea asked her questions like these, Ivonne had a reply ready.

"Andrea, your cousin Pilar wears glasses, doesn't she?" asked Ivonne. "Well, not *everyone* wears glasses, but Pilar does. She is a little different, but it's not her fault and it is not in a bad way at all. You like Pilar's glasses, don't you? Well, you have diabetes and not *everyone* has diabetes, but it is not your fault and it is not a bad thing. It is just something you have to learn to live with, like Pilar is learning to get used to her glasses."

That straightforward explanation made a world of difference to Andrea. Her self-confidence surged and she has not doubted herself since. Now, Andrea and her siblings attend Carmen Salles School, a known and highly respected Catholic school located about 12 kilometres from their home. The distance does not daunt Ivonne or Carlos, because their number one priority is to provide the best for their children whenever they can.

"We are lucky. Because of my job, I have good insurance and I can afford to take care of Andrea and all her diabetes needs," says Carlos. "For example, the insulin pump is something new that Andrea has to get used to right now. Such a pump would be very expensive if I didn't have insurance. In fact, Andrea is learning to regulate her blood sugar in a different way, as she learns about the pump and the right dosage of insulin for her, so she is having a pretty hard time. But it's not too bad, and we are here to help her, so we are all lucky."

Carlos knows how costly diabetes care can be without proper insurance. Paying for insulin, strips for the glucometer that tests the blood sugar levels, medical check-ups and other expenses is a huge burden for some families. Carlos is therefore looking ahead and has provided a security net for his daughter when she grows up

"Ivonne and I have set up a special bank account for Andrea," explains Carlos. Every month, he deposits money into the account, saving it for Andrea if she should ever need it. "This means that she will always be able to take care of her diabetes on heir own and will not have to rely on anyone. That is what I want for her."

A FALSE ALARM

❚❚She had never fallen asleep! She was listening out for the phone call."

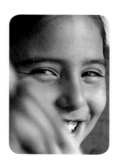

Carlos and Ivonne want Andrea to be well aware and well educated about diabetes and all it entails. As a result, they do not shelter her from the details of the complications that can occur if she ignores her diabetes.

Not long ago, Andrea went to one of her medical check-ups, which she goes to every three or four months. The tests were made at a laboratory in Cuernavaca.

"We were told that the X-rays that were taken of Andrea's liver and kidneys showed that she might have some serious problems with her kidneys," says Carlos. Andrea was only eight at the time and her parents were terrified. They rushed the lab results to Andrea's doctor in Mexico and waited for her opinion.

"Andrea was worried; she could sense our own worry, I think," says Carlos. "We had tried talking to her several times about the complications that may occur, but she never took it very seriously. Maybe she thought we were exaggerating so that she would not eat too many sweets. But when she saw us waiting by the phone that day, she was scared too."

When Andrea went to bed that night, she asked her parents to wake her as soon as the doctor called. Carlos admits that he never felt so scared in his life and tried hard to control himself, not wishing to show Ivonne the extent of his fear. "I had to be there for Ivonne, who was paralysed with worry. It was a hard day."

When the phone call finally came from Andrea's doctor, she had to explain that the lab in Cuernavaca had confused Andrea's results with those of another patient. Ivonne wept with relief and Carlos vowed to take Andrea to Mexico City from then on, whenever she needed medical attention or check-ups.

"Ivonne went into Andrea's room to wake her up and tell her everything was fine. We could not believe it when we saw that Andrea was already awake. She had never fallen asleep! She was listening out for the phone call. She finally understood the seriousness of what may happen to a person with diabetes who does not take proper care."

The false alarm accomplished what Carlos had been trying so hard to achieve: Andrea finally developed an awareness of the serious complications that may result from ignoring diabetes. Instead of remaining frightened by the incident, Andrea chose to learn from it. She displayed an admirable maturity for her age. Quietly and obediently, she sat still while her mother read aloud from a book on diabetes, the small exercises helping to answer some of the little girl's questions. She no longer laughs when her father tells her that failing eyesight and amputated limbs are serious consequences of neglecting one's diabetes.

And yet, Andrea is not worried. Living her life as fully as she can is all that matters to her; she refuses to waste time worrying or feeling sorry for herself. Already, the young girl considers herself lucky and blessed. She wants to make the most out of everything offered to her. The vibrant Andrea with the ever-present smile is living life to the brim.